THE *easy* diabetes COOKBOOK

Simple, Delicious Recipes
to Help You Balance Your Blood Sugars

mary ellen phipps

Registered Dietitian Nutritionist
and founder of Milk & Honey Nutrition®

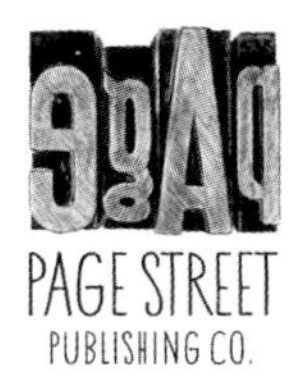

PAGE STREET
PUBLISHING CO.

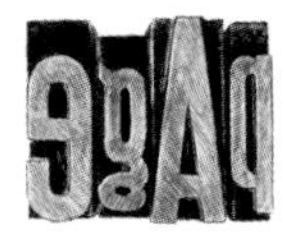

First published in 2021 by
Page Street Publishing Co.
27 Congress Street, Suite 105
Salem, MA 01970
www.pagestreetpublishing.com

Distributed by Macmillan, sales in Canada by The Canadian Manda Group.

25 24 23 22 21 1 2 3 4 5

ISBN-13: 978-1-64567-176-3
ISBN-10: 1-64567-176-3

Library of Congress Control Number: 2019957324

Cover and book design by Meghan Baskis for Page Street Publishing Co.
Photography by Lauren Kelp and Constance Mariena

Printed and bound in the United States

Page Street Publishing protects our planet by donating to nonprofits like The Trustees, which focuses on local land conservation.

To my parents for teaching me to go after my dreams,
to my husband for supporting my dreams,
and to my girls for always giving me a reason to dream bigger.

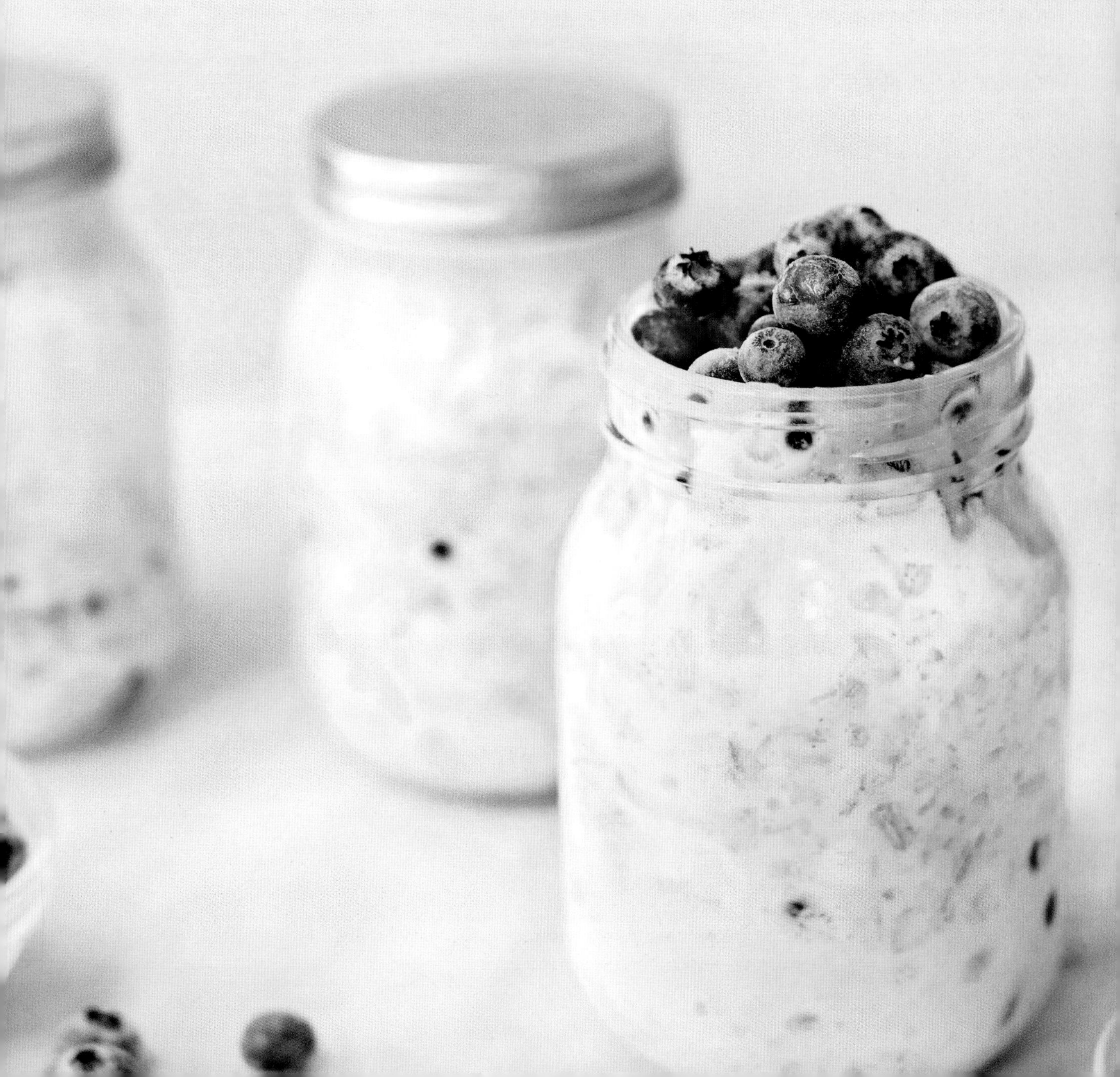

contents

introduction

Diabetes can hit you out of nowhere. It can be scary and overwhelming. It affects how you think, feel, act, move, eat, and so much more. It's a disease that not only affects the person diagnosed but also anyone close to that person.

Many people feel overwhelmed with the dietary and lifestyle changes they are told to make when they are first diagnosed. Most traditional advice involves cutting back on some foods or limiting certain nutrients. It can be a lot of information to take in. You may feel like diabetes is sucking the joy out of food—and possibly out of life. But if you have the right tools in place and know the scientific, proven strategies that make managing blood sugar levels easier, you'll be set up for success.

In this book, you'll learn another way to approach managing your blood sugar, bringing joy back to your kitchen and your life. You'll learn about the three key nutrients to add to your diet and how to use them to create some of the most delicious and blood sugar–friendly dishes you've ever tasted! A diagnosis of diabetes shouldn't mean an end to delicious food. I'll show you the tools you need and how to use them to feel confident in the kitchen again. In these pages, you'll find everything you need to know about eating to manage your blood sugars and living a healthy, less stressed, and more joyful life with diabetes.

But before we get to all the nutrition information and yummy recipes, let me tell you my story. You see, I'm just like you. I'm living with diabetes. I was diagnosed with type 1 diabetes at five years old. I have no memory of what life is like without diabetes. It's all I've ever known.

I was diagnosed in early August 1991, right before I was to start kindergarten. My mom, who also has type 1 diabetes, noticed that I had lost about 5 pounds (2.4 kg) without explanation, was suddenly wetting the bed again, and had developed a yeast infection. All of these are classic symptoms of the onset of type 1 diabetes. Sure enough—she tested my blood sugar, and it was well over 300 mg/dL (that's milligrams of glucose per deciliter of blood; typically, anything over 100 to 140, depending on the person's age and time of day, is considered abnormal). Like any concerned mom, she immediately called my pediatrician, who promptly told her she was just being paranoid since she had diabetes too. The doctor recommended that my mom should just keep an eye on me.

Thankfully, my mom rushed up to the pediatrician's office without an appointment and tested my blood sugar right there in front of the staff. Sure enough, still high. I had developed type 1 diabetes, and I spent five days at Cook Children's Medical Center in Fort Worth, Texas. I have vague memories of learning how to give myself shots, what foods contain carbohydrates, and what to do if my blood sugar went too high or too low.

Back then we didn't have all of the tools and medications to manage blood sugars that we do now. Both my mom and I had to eat pretty much the same things every day and maintain a consistent level of activity to help manage our blood sugars.

For the most part, I didn't mind—again, because I didn't really know any different. But it was the little things that got to me. For example, I had to scrape the icing off the cake at every birthday party I went to, and one time a mom who didn't know I had diabetes commented—to my face—what a strange kid I was for doing that. It's the first memory I have of feeling different and feeling that I wasn't "normal." And every day at school, I had to leave just before lunch to go to the nurse's office to test my blood sugar. I felt different and out of place.

When I was about ten years old, I was able to switch from older insulin formulas that required I eat the same things every day to a new, fast-acting insulin that allowed so much more freedom regarding what I ate and what I did each day. It was around this same time that I started to develop an interest in cooking and making food that worked for me.

My grandmother was one of the best cooks and bakers you could ever meet. She taught me how to make my first cheesecake, and there was no looking back. I fell in love with baking and learning how to make food that was blood sugar–friendly but also just as delicious as the "real thing." My Low-Sugar Blueberry Swirl Cheesecake (page 138) was inspired by my grandmother, so make sure to check it out if you enjoy cheesecake!

In college, I decided to major in nutrition once I found out I could actually make a career out of showing people how blood sugar–friendly foods can still taste amazing. Over the course of my career as a registered dietitian, I've realized there are two key things that help people living with diabetes successfully manage their blood sugars:

- They are educated on how food affects their own individual body.
- They truly enjoy the food they eat.

In the next section, we'll cover the three key nutrients that are crucial to managing blood sugars and should be the focus of all your meals and snacks. But it's important to remember that you are unique and should be treated as such. What works for you may not work for the next person, and vice versa. It's okay to experiment a little and figure out what foods your blood sugars respond well to and what foods they don't. I encourage you to use what you learn in this book and apply it to your own situation. And always talk to your doctor or dietitian if you have any questions.

Mary Ellen Phipps

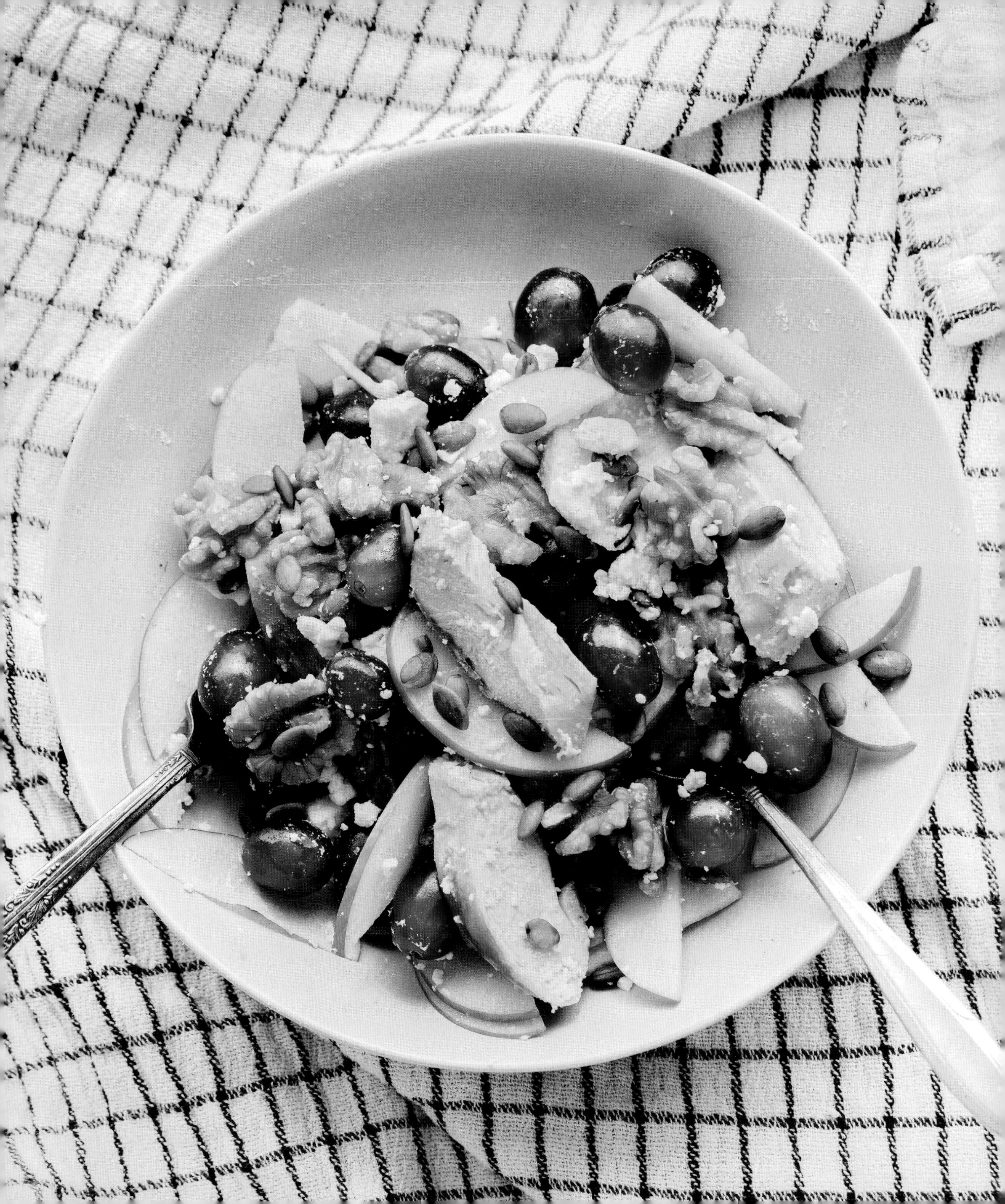

fat, fiber, and protein

THE THREE KEYS TO BALANCING BLOOD SUGARS

What if managing your diabetes revolved around what to add to your diet instead of what to take away? What if the focus was on nourishing your body the right way and not on depriving or restricting yourself? Fat, fiber, and protein are all nutrients—and key tools—that add both flavor and satisfaction to dishes while also helping nourish your body and manage blood sugar levels. They all have the ability to delay your body's absorption of carbohydrates, both after a meal and throughout the day.

Having fat, fiber, and protein present in a meal means it will take your body longer to digest your food, and thus longer for nutrients to get absorbed into your bloodstream. This includes carbohydrates, and this is a good thing!

Delayed absorption of carbohydrates means several things:

- A more consistent, steadier supply of energy after you eat.
- A feeling of fullness and satisfaction for longer periods of time.
- A steadier blood sugar response after you eat (e.g., no sugar crashes).

If you eat carbohydrates by themselves, they get processed by your body very quickly—this means an instant supply of energy, but it also means a rapid rise in blood sugar levels, which we don't want.

What Happens When You Eat

Even people without diabetes will see a rise in their blood sugar levels after they eat. This is a normal response by your body. Your GI tract will break down the food you eat into specific nutrients. As you might already know, carbohydrates are broken down into glucose (i.e., sugar) and are absorbed into your bloodstream. This is why we refer to glucose in the bloodstream as blood sugar levels. Glucose is vital to your body's cells and is essential for thousands of processes that happen in the body.

At this point, the pancreas of someone without diabetes will release a hormone called insulin into the bloodstream. Insulin acts like a key that unlocks the door to each of your body's cells, allowing the glucose to go inside and be used for energy. Without adequate amounts of insulin, extra glucose builds up in the bloodstream and can have negative health impacts over time.

If you have prediabetes, type 2 diabetes, or gestational diabetes:

- your pancreas is struggling to keep up and not able to produce enough insulin for the amount of carbohydrates you eat; or
- the insulin your pancreas is producing is not as effective as it used to be, and your pancreas has to produce more insulin than it used to.

If you have type 1 diabetes, your pancreas is not able to produce any insulin, and you must inject insulin from an outside source, such as insulin pens or an exterior insulin pump.

In both of these situations, whether it's the insulin coming from your own pancreas that is delayed or less effective or insulin being injected from an outside source, one thing is the same: The insulin does not work as fast as your body thinks it does. When you live with any type of diabetes, wherever the insulin is coming from, it cannot keep up with the rapid rise in blood sugar that happens when you eat carbohydrates by themselves.

Think of the rise and fall of blood sugars as an intense and scary roller coaster you've seen or ridden at an amusement park, with lots of steep ups and downs. That's what your blood sugar levels look like if there are no "buffers" like fat, fiber, and protein in the food you eat.

When we add fat, fiber, and protein to our meals, we get a steadier rise and fall. Think of the kiddie roller coasters meant for toddlers and young children, with flatter and more gradual hills. Fat, fiber, and protein literally act as buffers to blunt the rise and fall in blood sugar levels. Fat, fiber, and protein delay the absorption of carbohydrates and allow the insulin to "catch up" with the level of glucose in the blood, thus avoiding any steep ascents and descents.

Think about the last time you ate a piece of candy or had something like syrup or honey. Those are very rapid-acting carbohydrates that cause a quick rise in blood sugar and often a subsequent "crash." The term *sugar crash*, though exaggerated at times, is a legitimate phenomenon: Your blood sugar rises very quickly and the insulin can't quite keep up to get those glucose molecules into your body's cells fast enough. By the time it does, there is an equally quick fall in blood sugar levels back down to normal. That rapid fall is a sugar crash.

Let's look at an example of fat, fiber, and protein slowing things down. If you eat a plain piece of white bread with nothing on it, your body is able to process that piece of bread pretty quickly. It will be gone from your stomach and on its way to being absorbed by your GI tract within an hour. This means two things:

- You'll be hungry again soon, leaving you unsatisfied and looking for more food.
- The carbohydrates in that piece of bread are broken down quickly and raise your blood sugars fast.

Now, let's say you add some butter to that white bread. There's still not much fiber or protein in it, but you have added a small amount of fat. This fat will slow down your body's processing of that piece of bread. It takes your GI tract longer to process fat. That one piece of white bread will now keep you fuller for a little bit longer and raise your blood sugar at a slightly slower rate—but not by much.

But if you swap that piece of white bread for a piece of whole-grain bread (adding fiber and protein), and add some avocado on top (adding healthy fat and fiber), you'll have an even better option! This piece of higher-fiber and higher-fat avocado toast gets absorbed more slowly, keeping you full and satisfied for longer and those post-meal blood sugars nice and steady.

ONE EXCEPTION TO REMEMBER

The one time you actually want to avoid fat, fiber, and protein is when you are treating low blood sugars. Your doctor or diabetes educator has likely told you to avoid these things when your blood sugars are low. Carbohydrates in isolation raise blood sugar levels very quickly and a period of low blood sugars is usually the only time we actually want that to happen.

Putting It into Practice

All of the recipes in this book use some combination of fat, fiber, and protein to help promote stable and balanced post-meal and post-snack blood sugar levels. Like my Blueberry Cheesecake Overnight Oats (page 16), they not only taste amazing but the cream cheese and oats (offering fat and fiber, respectively) help buffer any potential blood sugar spike that would arise from the maple syrup. And my Coconut-Crusted Chicken Tenders (page 39) use coconut flour as a lower-glycemic alternative to flours traditionally used to bread meats, thus avoiding any potential blood sugar spikes altogether. Coconut flour has fewer carbohydrates, more fat and more fiber than traditional white flour.

Making the recipes in this book will help you manage your diabetes, boost your energy, and most importantly, give you more satisfaction and less stress about the food you are eating!

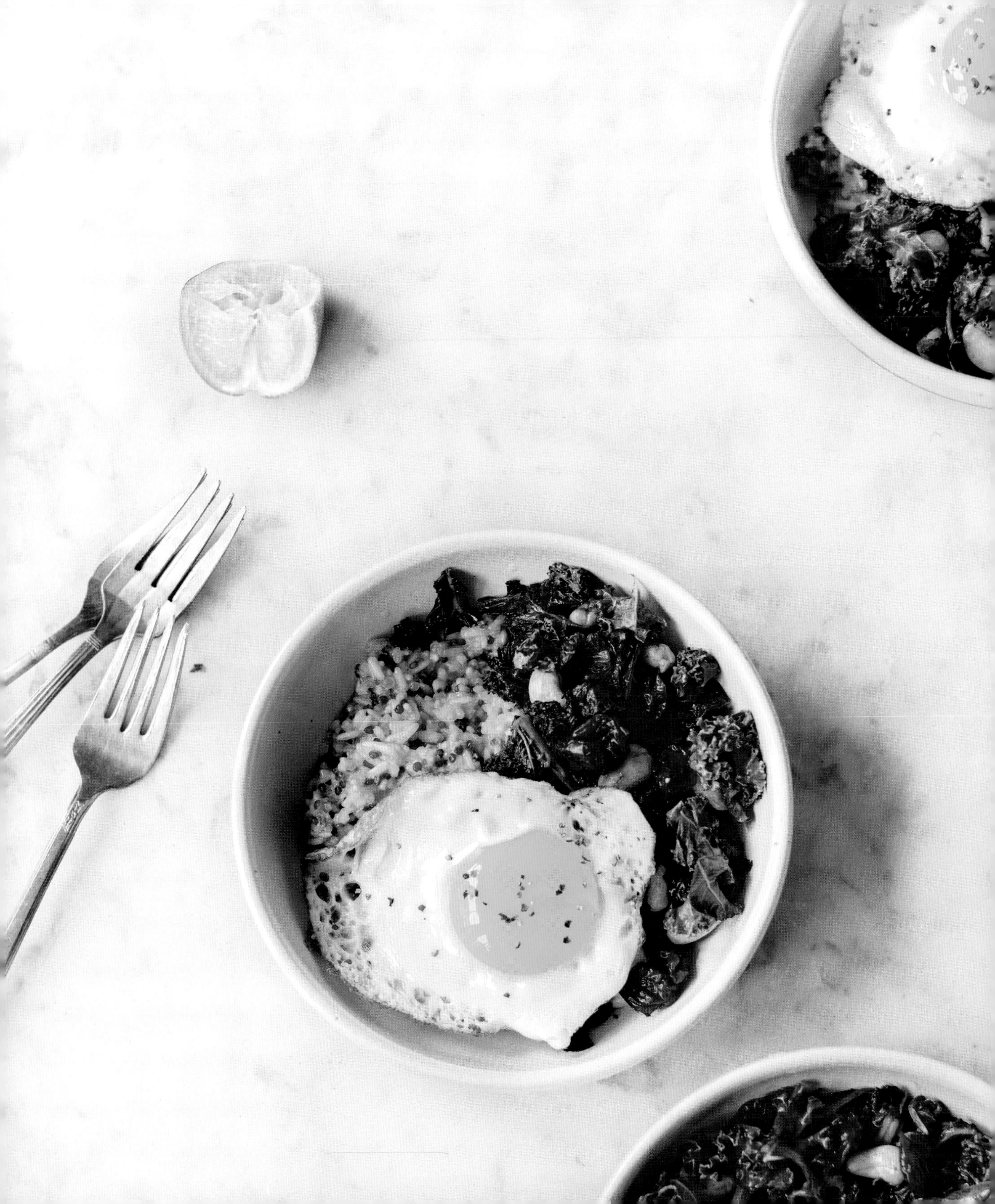

deliciously satisfying and nourishing recipes

Get ready for some delicious recipes packed with fat, fiber, and protein! Next to each recipe you'll notice some categorizations. Here's what they all mean:

- **Gluten-Free:** Many people with type 1 diabetes may also have celiac disease or a non-celiac gluten sensitivity. Recipes with this label are made with gluten-free ingredients.
- **High Fiber:** Fiber is great for keeping your gut healthy and keeping you full and satisfied. We also know that a diet high in fiber has been linked to reduced complications from diseases like diabetes. Recipes with this label have 5 or more grams of fiber per serving.
- **Low Carb:** While a completely low-carbohydrate diet is not necessary to balance blood sugars, sometimes a lower-carbohydrate version of a recipe is a better option. Recipes with this label have 15 or fewer grams of carbohydrates per serving.
- **No Added Sugar:** While sugar is sugar, it's important to note that naturally occurring sugars also typically come with vitamins, minerals, and fiber, like the sugars in fruit. Recipes with this label have no added sugar, and any sweetness comes from naturally occurring sugars.
- **Protein Packed:** As I mentioned before, it's important for people with diabetes to eat quality protein sources throughout the day. Recipes with this label have 20 or more grams of protein per serving.
- **Sodium Aware:** Many people with diabetes may also have hypertension or may have been told to limit their sodium intake. Recipes with this label have 250 or fewer milligrams of sodium per serving. (Note: This is different from foods labeled as "low sodium" that you've likely seen at the grocery store. "Low sodium" refers to foods with 140 milligrams of sodium or less per serving.)
- **Vegan:** People living with diabetes may benefit from a plant-based diet or just simply from eating more plants. Recipes with this label are made with completely plant-based ingredients.

NOTE ON NUTRITION FACTS

The nutrition facts presented in this book are estimates only. The brands you use and product types you choose can change the nutritional information presented. To obtain the most accurate nutritional information, you should calculate the nutritional information with the actual ingredients you use.

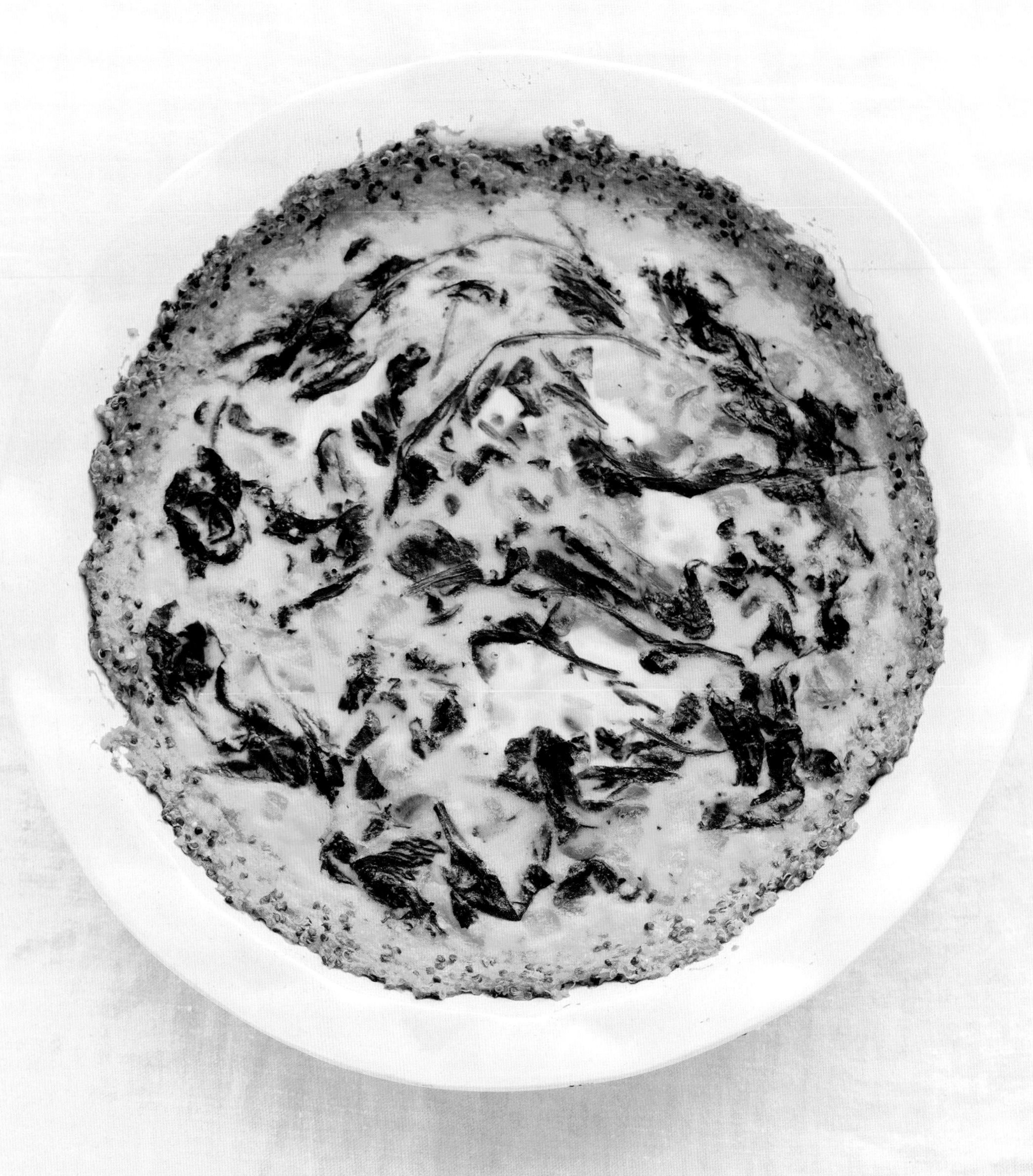

blood sugar–balancing breakfasts

ENERGIZING EATS TO START YOUR DAY

Starting your day with a blood sugar–balancing breakfast is essential for keeping blood sugars stable throughout the day. Most people, whether they have diabetes or not, are more insulin resistant in the morning due to naturally occurring hormones that help our bodies get going at the start of the day. When you have diabetes, this insulin resistance can be amplified even more. To combat this, it is ideal to make sure you have an adequate balance of fat, fiber, and protein in your breakfast.

There are many foods that not only taste delicious but can also be a part of a blood sugar–friendly breakfast because of their fat, fiber, and protein content, as well as their lower sugar content.

Fat sources I recommend are:

- Avocado
- Nuts and seeds
- Nut butter

Protein sources I recommend are:

- Eggs
- Greek yogurt
- Quinoa

Fiber sources I recommend are:

- Berries
- Veggies
- Whole-grain breads

Some of the recipes in this chapter can be made the morning of, like my Chocolate-Cherry Smoothie (page 19), and some are ideal for prepping on the weekend so you can grab them and get out the door on weekday mornings, like my Grain-Free Coconut and Almond Waffles (page 32).

blueberry cheesecake overnight oats

These Blueberry Cheesecake Overnight Oats are a perfect way to start your day and keep your blood sugars on track. The cream cheese in this recipe adds fat and a creaminess that makes the dish more satisfying and friendlier to your blood sugars. The lemon zest and vanilla extract add flavorful sweetness without actually adding much sugar.

gluten-free | high fiber | sodium aware | yield: 4 servings

4 oz (113 g) cream cheese

½ cup (100 g) plain Greek yogurt

2 cups (480 ml) unsweetened almond milk

2 tbsp (30 ml) pure maple syrup

Zest of 1 medium lemon

1 tbsp (15 ml) pure vanilla extract

2 cups (300 g) frozen blueberries

2 cups (160 g) gluten-free rolled oats

Set out four (12-oz [340-ml]) glass jars with their lids.

In a large mixing bowl, combine the cream cheese, yogurt, almond milk, maple syrup, lemon zest, and vanilla. Whisk the ingredients together until they are smooth. Or, for an extra smooth texture, combine the ingredients in a food processor. Set the mixing bowl aside.

Add ½ cup (75 g) of blueberries to each jar. Then add ½ cup (40 g) of oats to each jar on top of the blueberries.

Divide the cream cheese mixture evenly between the four jars.

Secure the lid on each jar, and shake each jar vigorously to combine the ingredients. Place the jars in the refrigerator overnight. Then, just pull a jar of your overnight oats out the next morning, top it off with some extra blueberries, and enjoy!

STORAGE: Each jar will keep in the refrigerator for up to 5 days if sealed tightly and unopened.

TIP: This recipe can be enjoyed warm too. After the overnight oats have set overnight in your refrigerator, just remove the lid, place the jar in the microwave, and heat the oats on high for 30 to 45 seconds, to your desired temperature.

Estimated Nutrition Facts per Serving: 412 calories; 53 g carbs; 8 g fiber; 16 g sugar (6 g added sugar); 12 g protein; 16 g fat (7.5 g saturated fat); 207 mg sodium

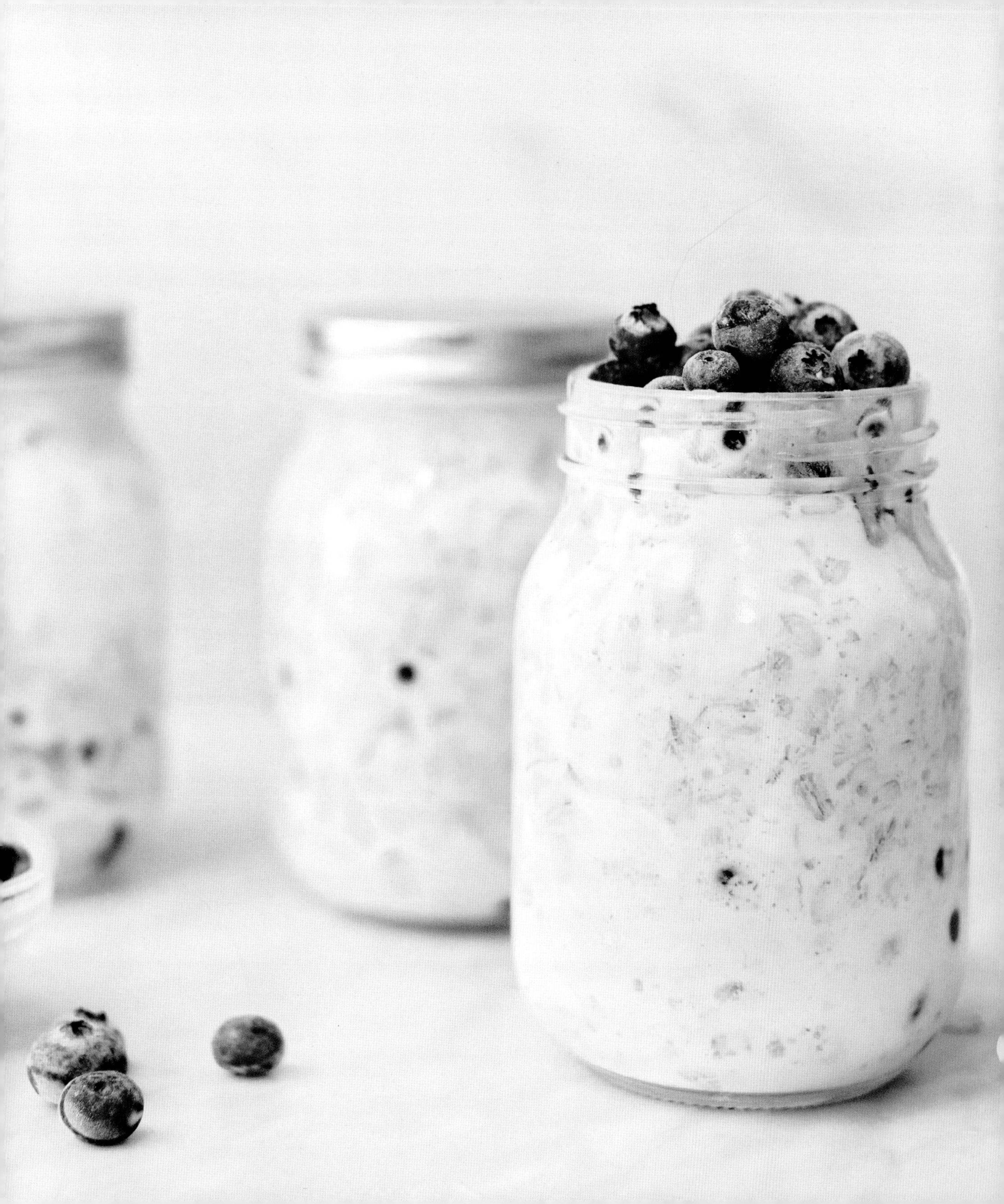

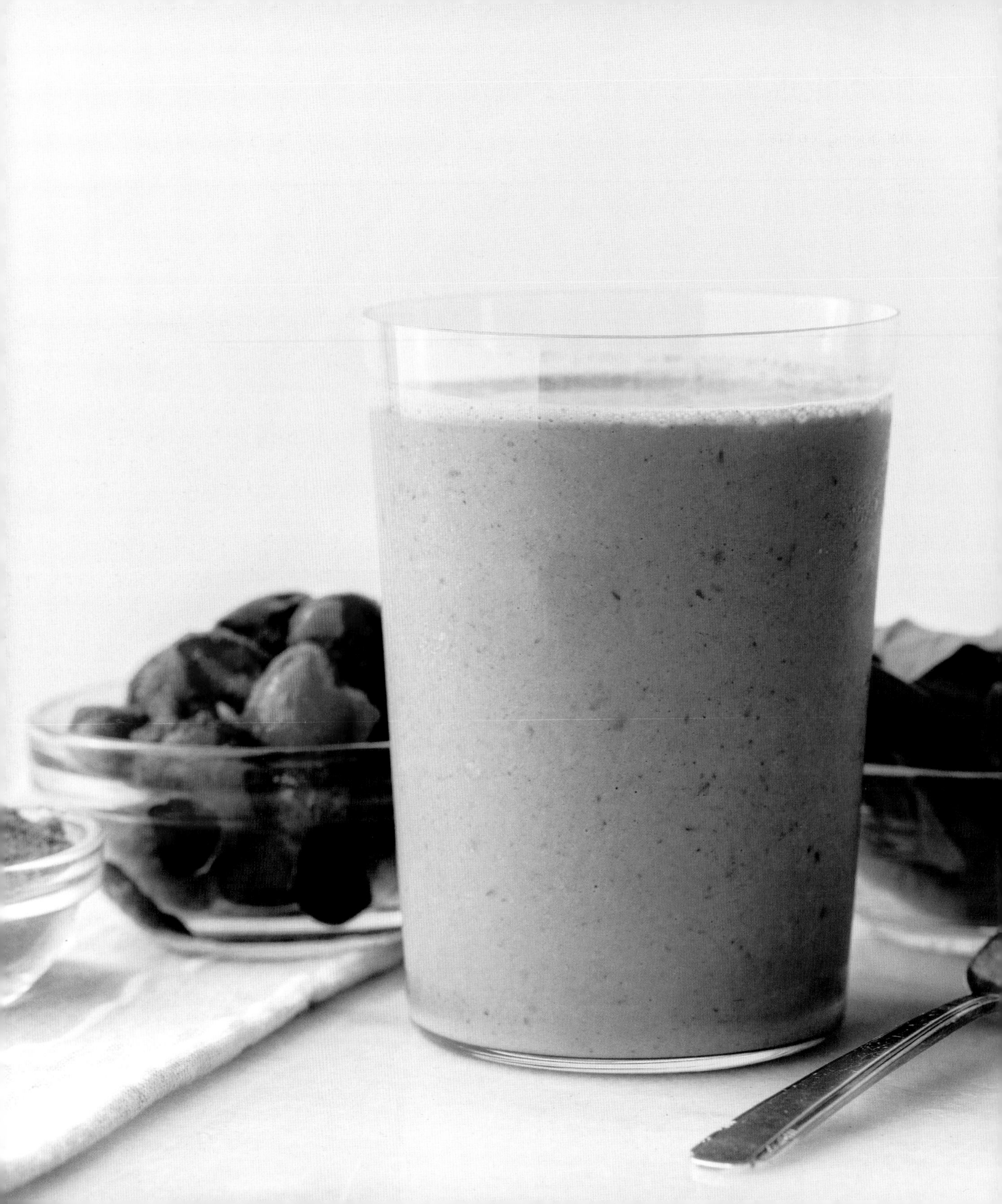

chocolate-cherry smoothie

It's like having ice cream for breakfast with this thick and creamy smoothie! I love having a smoothie in the morning for a quick and nutritious breakfast that helps keep my blood sugars balanced until lunchtime. Fiber from the cherries and spinach, fat from the almond butter, and protein from the Greek yogurt will all help keep you full, satisfied, and energized.

gluten-free | high fiber | no added sugar | protein packed | sodium aware | yield: 1 serving

1 cup (154 g) frozen cherries

½ cup (45 g) frozen spinach or 1 cup (30 g) fresh spinach

1 tbsp (15 g) almond butter

1 tbsp (6 g) unsweetened cocoa powder

¾ cup (150 g) plain nonfat Greek yogurt

In a high-power blender, combine the cherries, spinach, almond butter, cocoa powder, and yogurt. Blend the ingredients for 30 to 45 seconds, until they are smooth.

STORAGE: This smoothie should be eaten immediately. To prep it ahead of time, add the cherries, spinach, almond butter, and cocoa powder to a freezer-safe container or bag, freeze, and blend the frozen ingredients with the yogurt the morning of, according to the directions.

Estimated Nutrition Facts per Serving: 331 calories; 33 g carbs; 8 g fiber; 20 g sugar; 25 g protein; 11 g fat (1 g saturated fat); 125 mg sodium

sunrise smoothie bowl

Smoothie bowls are a trendy juice bar staple, but the average store-bought version is high in sugar and lacking in fiber. This homemade smoothie bowl boasts over half of your daily fiber needs and 17 grams of protein. Fiber and protein make this smoothie bowl an actual meal that will keep you full and your blood sugars steady!

gluten-free | high fiber | no added sugar | sodium aware | yield: 1 serving

½ cup (63 g) frozen raspberries

½ cup (72 g) frozen strawberries

½ large banana

½ cup (50 g) cauliflower florets

½ cup (100 g) plain nonfat Greek yogurt

Water, as needed

1 tbsp (5 g) unsweetened coconut flakes

2 tbsp (14 g) coarsely chopped walnuts

In a high-power blender, combine the raspberries, strawberries, banana, cauliflower, and yogurt. Blend the ingredients until they are smooth, adding water as needed to reach the desired consistency.

Pour the smoothie into a bowl and top it with the coconut flakes and walnuts.

STORAGE: Enjoy this smoothie bowl immediately. To prepare it ahead of time, add the raspberries, strawberries, banana, and cauliflower to a freezer-safe container or bag and freeze. Add yogurt and blend the smoothie bowl and add toppings the morning of, according to the directions.

Estimated Nutrition Facts per Serving: 336 calories; 44 g carbs; 12 g fiber; 21 g sugar; 17 g protein; 14 g fat (4 g saturated fat); 69 mg sodium

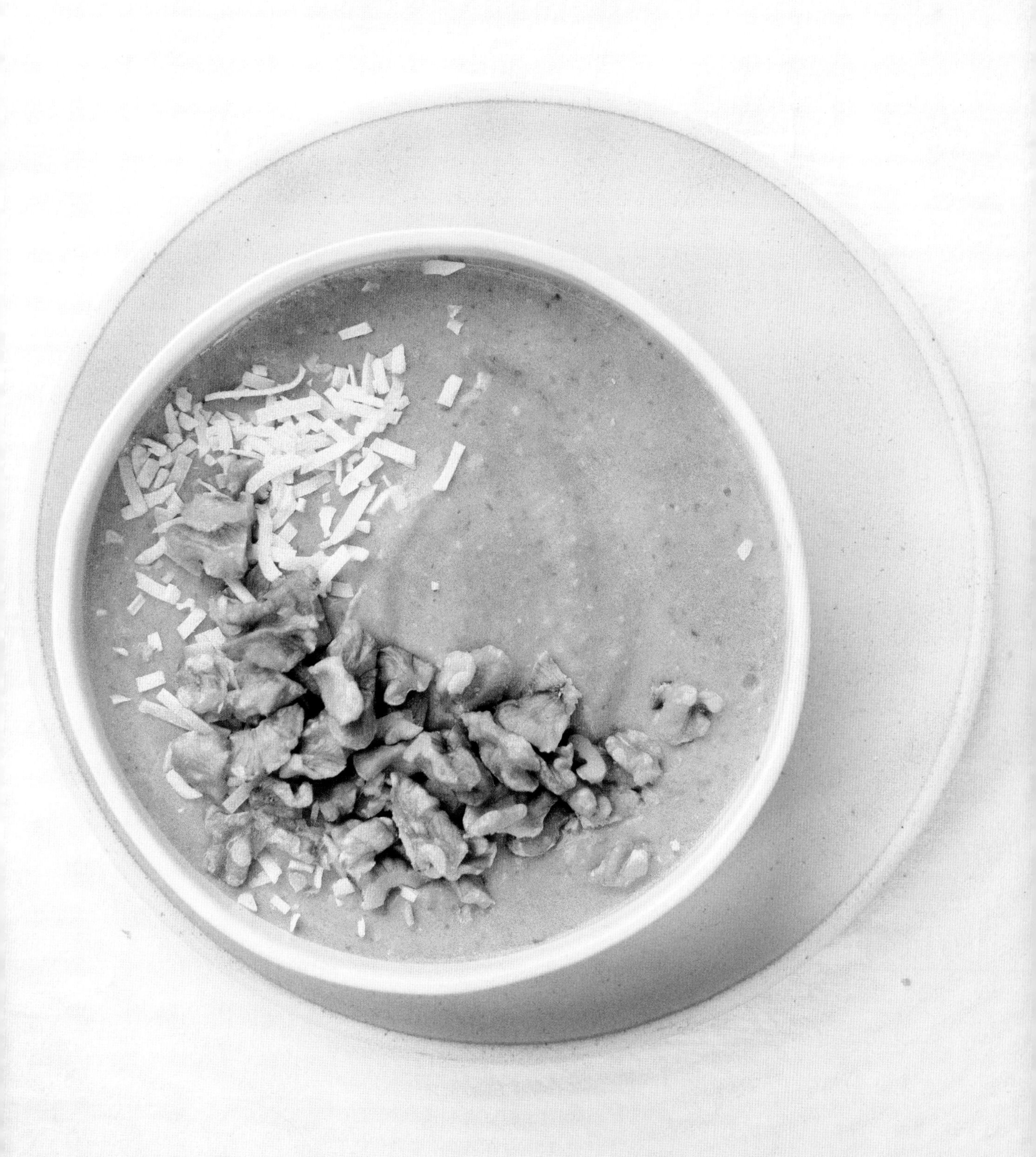

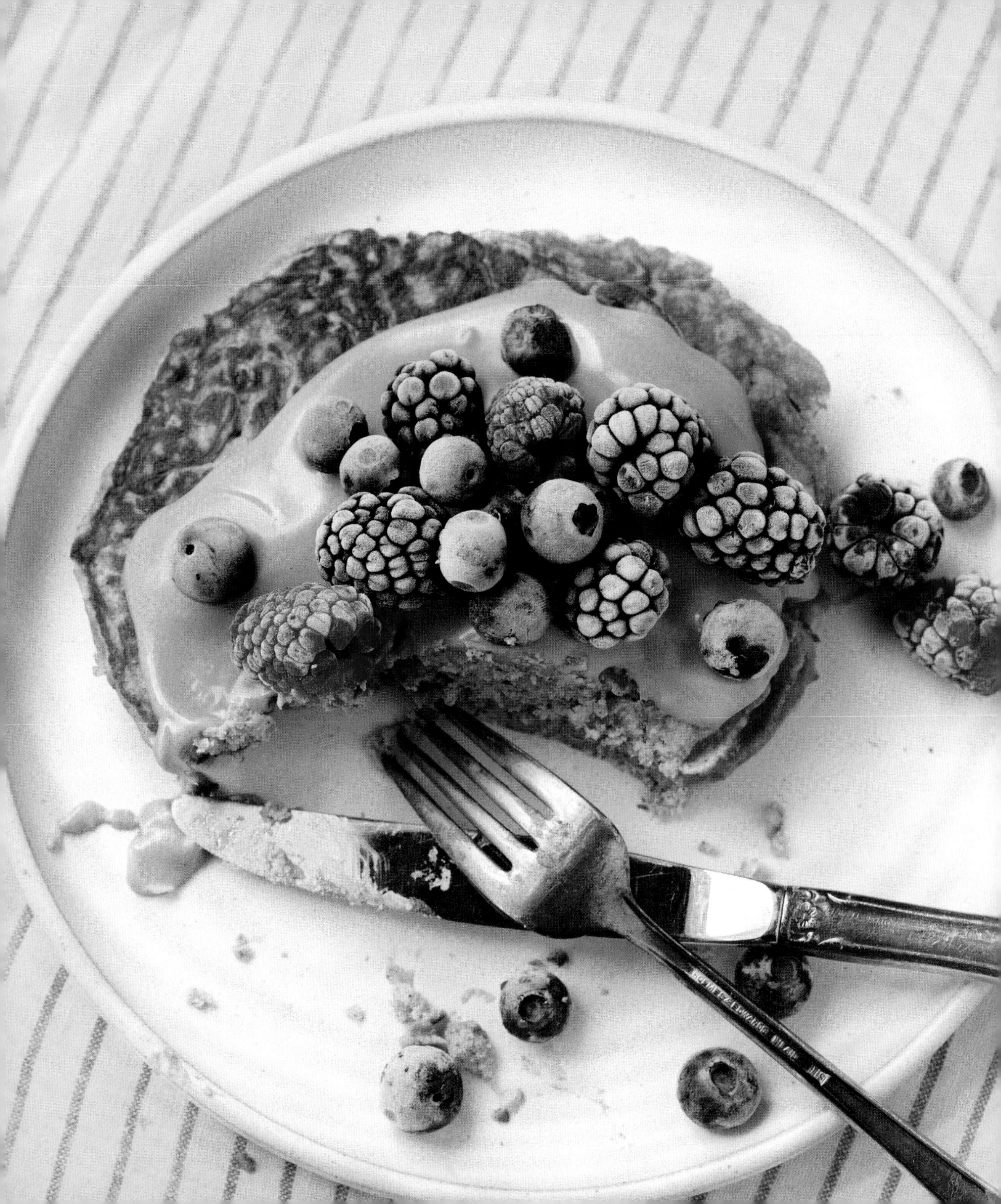

banana protein pancakes

It's important to start each day with a hearty breakfast, and these Banana Protein Pancakes are a perfect way to do just that! These pancakes offer a higher protein and fiber content than traditional pancakes, making them a fantastic option for balancing blood sugars. Finish them off with some drizzled peanut butter and fresh or frozen fruit for the perfect blood sugar–friendly meal.

high fiber | no added sugar | sodium aware | yield: 4 servings

Cooking oil spray, as needed (optional)

2 medium bananas

1 large avocado, mashed

4 large eggs

½ cup (120 ml) egg whites

2 tsp (10 ml) pure vanilla extract

2 tsp (8 g) baking powder

½ cup (50 g) whole-wheat flour

½ cup (56 g) coconut flour

1 tsp ground cinnamon

All-natural peanut butter, as needed (see Tip)

Thawed frozen fruit, as needed

Heat a large nonstick skillet over medium heat until it is very hot. Spray the skillet lightly with the cooking oil spray (if using).

In a large bowl, mash the bananas. Whisk in the avocado, eggs, egg whites, and vanilla. Add the baking powder, whole-wheat flour, coconut flour, and cinnamon. Mix the batter until the ingredients are well combined.

Using a ¼-cup (60-ml) measuring cup, scoop the batter onto the skillet. Gently spread out the batter to create a circle if needed. Cook the pancakes for 3 minutes, flip them, and cook them for 2 to 3 minutes on the opposite side. The pancakes will be golden brown and ready to enjoy!

Drizzle the pancakes with the peanut butter and place the fruit on top just prior to serving.

STORAGE: If you will not be eating all of the pancakes right away, freeze them for an easy breakfast to pop in the toaster on busy mornings.

TIP: Be sure to buy an all-natural peanut butter with no added salt or sugar.

Estimated Nutrition Facts per Serving: 357 calories; 39 g carbs; 12 g fiber; 9 g sugar; 15 g protein; 17 g fat (5 g saturated fat); 158 mg sodium

peaches and cream yogurt bowl

This recipe takes the typical peach pie and transforms it into a delicious diabetes-friendly breakfast bowl! This yogurt bowl is high in fiber, high in protein, and naturally sweet. You can also get creative and swap in your favorite fruit and nut butter.

gluten-free | high fiber | protein packed | sodium aware | yield: 1 serving

6 oz (170 g) plain Greek yogurt

½ tsp pure vanilla extract

½ tsp ground cinnamon

1 medium peach, sliced to desired thickness, or 1 cup (250 g) frozen sliced peaches

1 tbsp (15 g) almond butter

1 tsp honey (optional)

In a small bowl, stir together the yogurt, vanilla, and cinnamon. Add the peach slices and drizzle the yogurt bowl with the almond butter and honey (if using).

STORAGE: This yogurt bowl is best enjoyed shortly after you make it.

TIP: If you are using frozen peaches, you can leave them frozen or defrost them to room temperature. Either way they'll taste delicious!

Estimated Nutrition Facts per Serving without Honey: 361 calories; 27 g carbs; 6 g fiber; 21 g sugar; 24 g protein; 19 g fat (2 g saturated fat); 91 mg sodium

Estimated Nutrition Facts per Serving with Honey: 381 calories; 33 g carbs; 6 g fiber; 26 g sugar; 24 g protein; 19 g fat (2 g saturated fat); 91 mg sodium

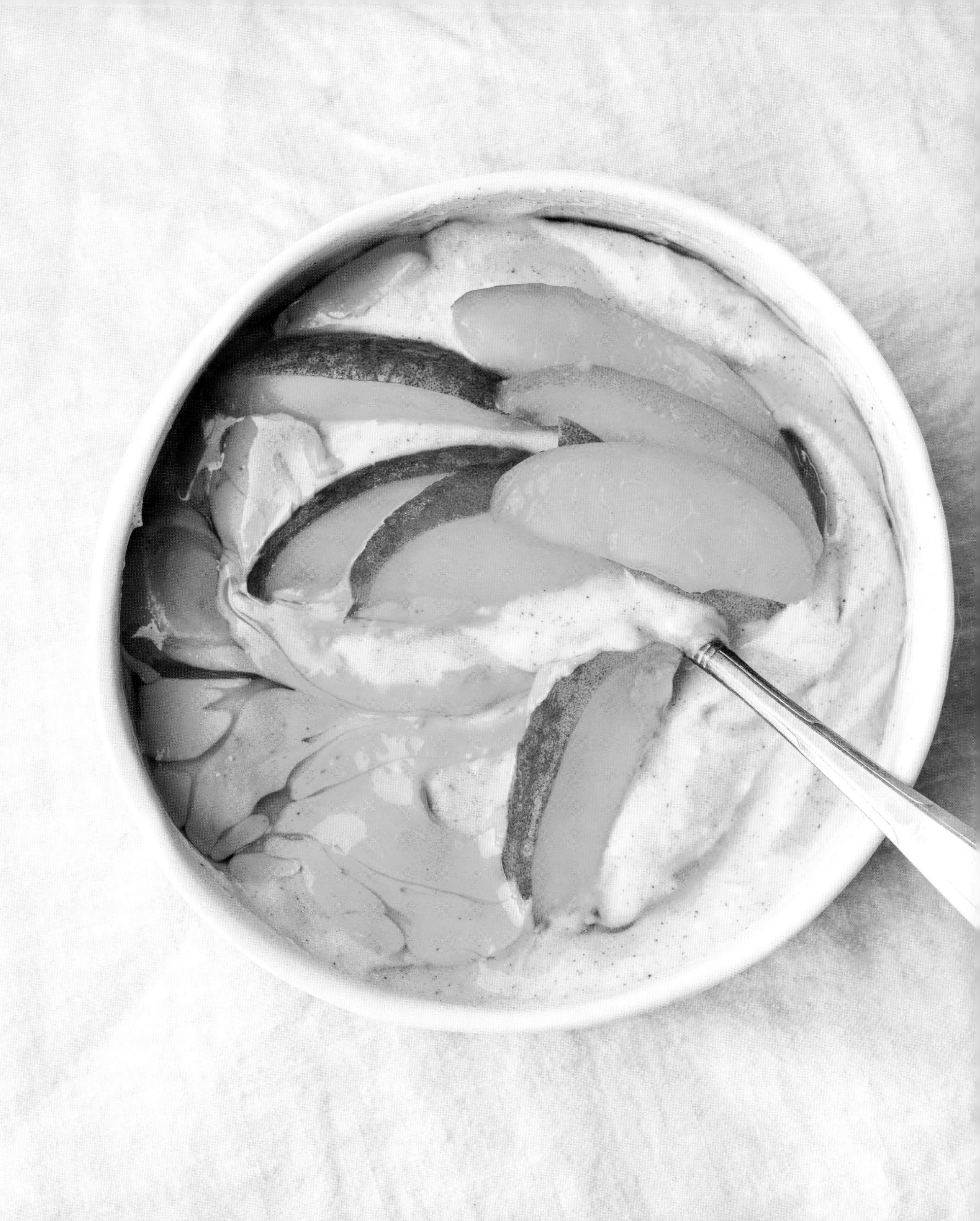

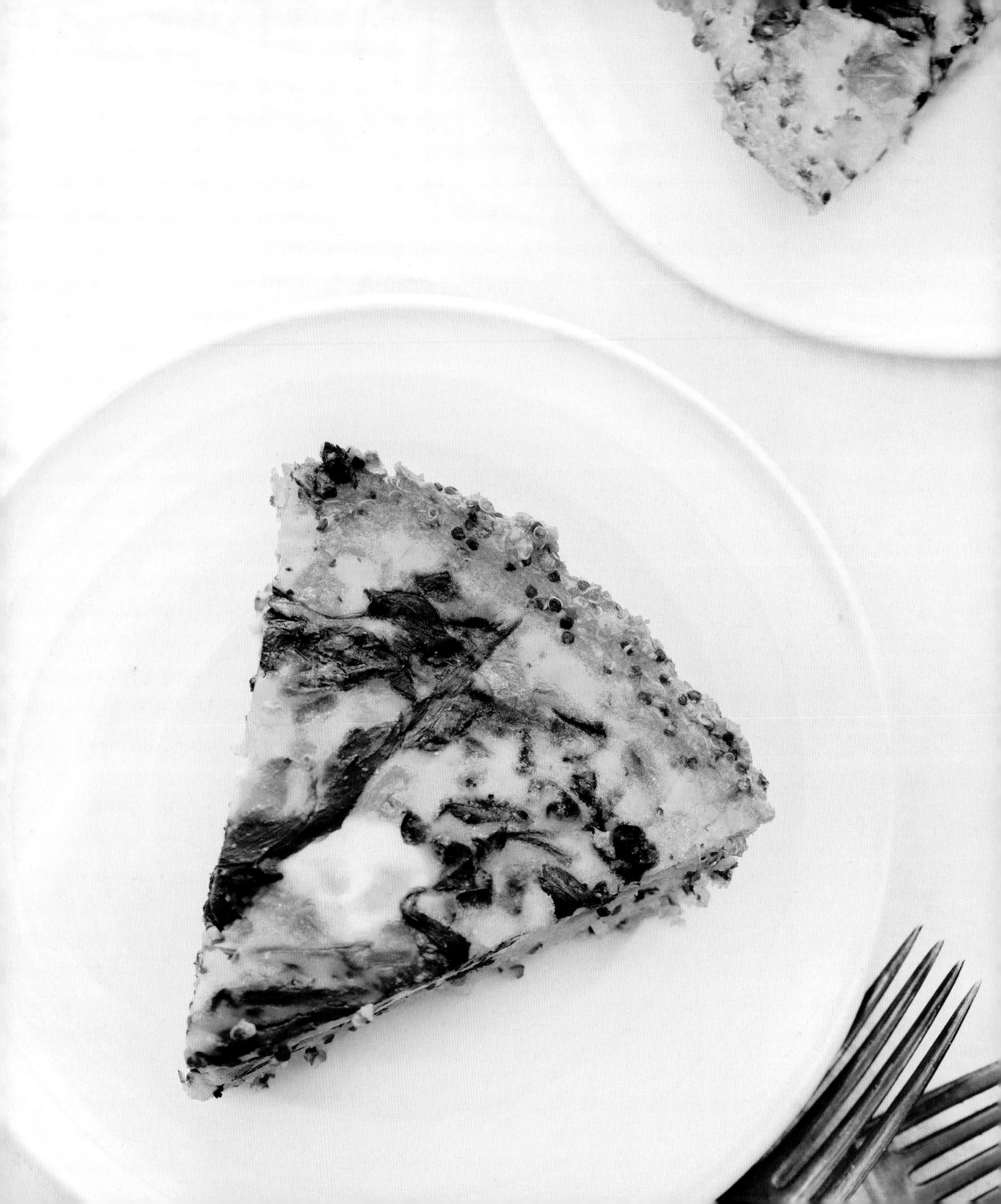

cheesy quinoa-crusted spinach frittata

This recipe will make weekday breakfasts a breeze. Prep it on the weekend and have a blood sugar–balancing, gourmet breakfast ready to go for the week! The quinoa crust adds more fiber and protein than a traditional pastry crust to better stabilize blood sugars and fuel your morning.

gluten-free | no added sugar | protein packed | yield: 4 servings

1 cup (170 g) uncooked quinoa

Cooking oil spray, as needed

½ cup (120 ml) egg whites

¾ cup (90 g) shredded Cheddar cheese

½ tbsp (8 ml) cooking oil of choice

½ medium yellow onion, diced

5 oz (142 g) baby spinach

6 large eggs

⅔ cup (160 ml) 2% milk

½ tsp mustard powder

½ tsp sea salt

¼ tsp black pepper

In a medium pot, cook the quinoa according to the package instructions. Set the quinoa aside to cool in the pot.

Preheat the oven to 375°F (191°C). Spray a 9-inch (23-cm) pie dish with the cooking oil spray.

Once the quinoa has cooled, add the egg whites and Cheddar cheese, stirring to combine the ingredients. Carefully press the quinoa mixture into the prepared pie dish. Bake the crust for 15 minutes. Remove the crust from the oven and allow it to cool.

While the crust is baking, heat the oil in a medium skillet over medium heat. Add the onion and spinach and sauté them for 10 to 15 minutes, until the onion is translucent and the spinach is wilted. Set the vegetables aside to cool.

Meanwhile, combine the eggs, milk, mustard powder, salt, and black pepper in a medium bowl and whisk to combine the ingredients.

Add the sautéed vegetables to the crust and spread them into an even layer. Pour the egg mixture over the vegetables.

Return the frittata to the oven and bake it for 35 to 40 minutes, or until the eggs have set in the middle.

STORAGE: This frittata will keep, covered, in an airtight container in the refrigerator for up to 5 days.

Estimated Nutrition Facts per Serving: 414 calories; 33 g carbs; 4 g fiber; 4 g sugar; 26 g protein; 19 g fat (8 g saturated fat); 624 mg sodium

crustless potato, spinach, and mushroom quiche

Crispy potatoes take the place of a traditional pastry crust for this nutrient-packed quiche, while balsamic-roasted mushrooms, sun-dried tomatoes, and spinach add flavor and fiber to every bite. Be sure to keep the skins on the potatoes for an even bigger fiber boost that keeps blood sugars nice and steady!

gluten-free | no added sugar | protein packed | sodium aware | yield: 4 servings

8 oz (227 g) yellow potatoes, thinly sliced

1 tbsp (15 ml) olive oil

2 tsp (2 g) dried thyme, divided

1 tsp dried rosemary

10 oz (283 g) button mushrooms, coarsely chopped

1 tsp balsamic vinegar

2 cups (60 g) baby spinach

6 large eggs

2 cups (480 ml) 1% milk

2 oz (57 g) goat cheese, crumbled

½ cup (28 g) julienned sun-dried tomatoes (see Tip)

Preheat the oven to 375°F (191°C).

In a large bowl, toss the potatoes with the oil, 1 teaspoon of the thyme, and rosemary. Arrange the potatoes on the bottom of a large oven-safe skillet or baking dish. Bake the potatoes for 10 to 15 minutes, or until they soften and start to crisp. Do not turn off the oven.

Meanwhile, combine the remaining 1 teaspoon of thyme and the mushrooms in a large skillet over medium-high heat. Cook the mushrooms for about 5 minutes, or until the mushrooms are brown and most of their liquid has evaporated. Stir in the vinegar. Add the spinach and cook it for 3 to 4 minutes, stirring constantly, until it is wilted. Remove the mushrooms and spinach from the heat and set them aside.

In a large bowl, whisk together the eggs and milk. Add the mushroom and spinach mixture, goat cheese, and sun-dried tomatoes. Pour the mixture into the potato-lined skillet and bake the quiche for 25 minutes, or until the eggs are set and no longer runny in the center.

STORAGE: This quiche will keep in an airtight container in the refrigerator for up to 5 days.

TIP: Be sure to purchase packaged julienned sun-dried tomatoes, not the jarred variety that are packed in oil.

Estimated Nutrition Facts per Serving: 322 calories; 25 g carbs; 3 g fiber; 12 g sugar; 22 g protein; 16 g fat (6 g saturated fat); 218 mg sodium

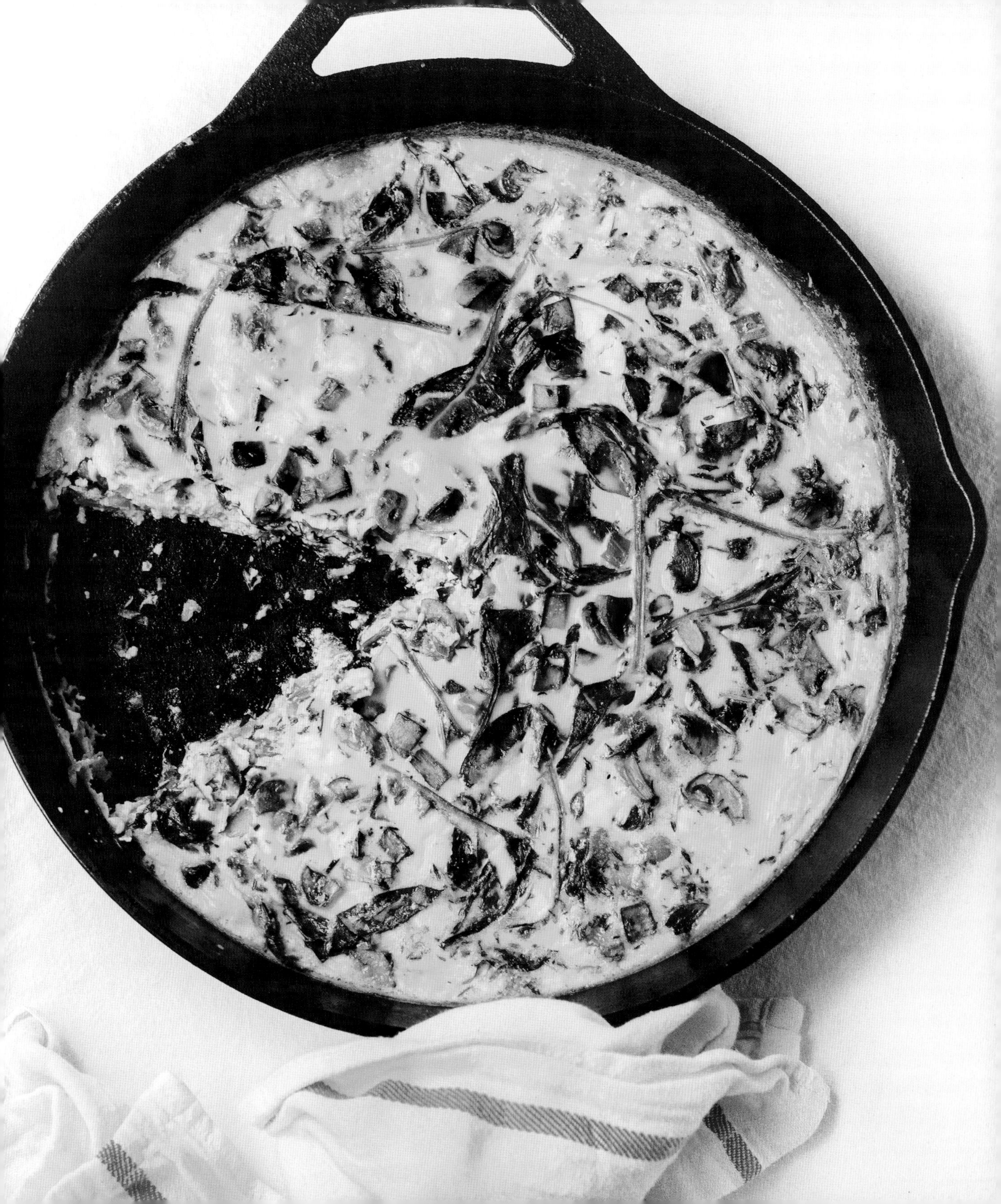

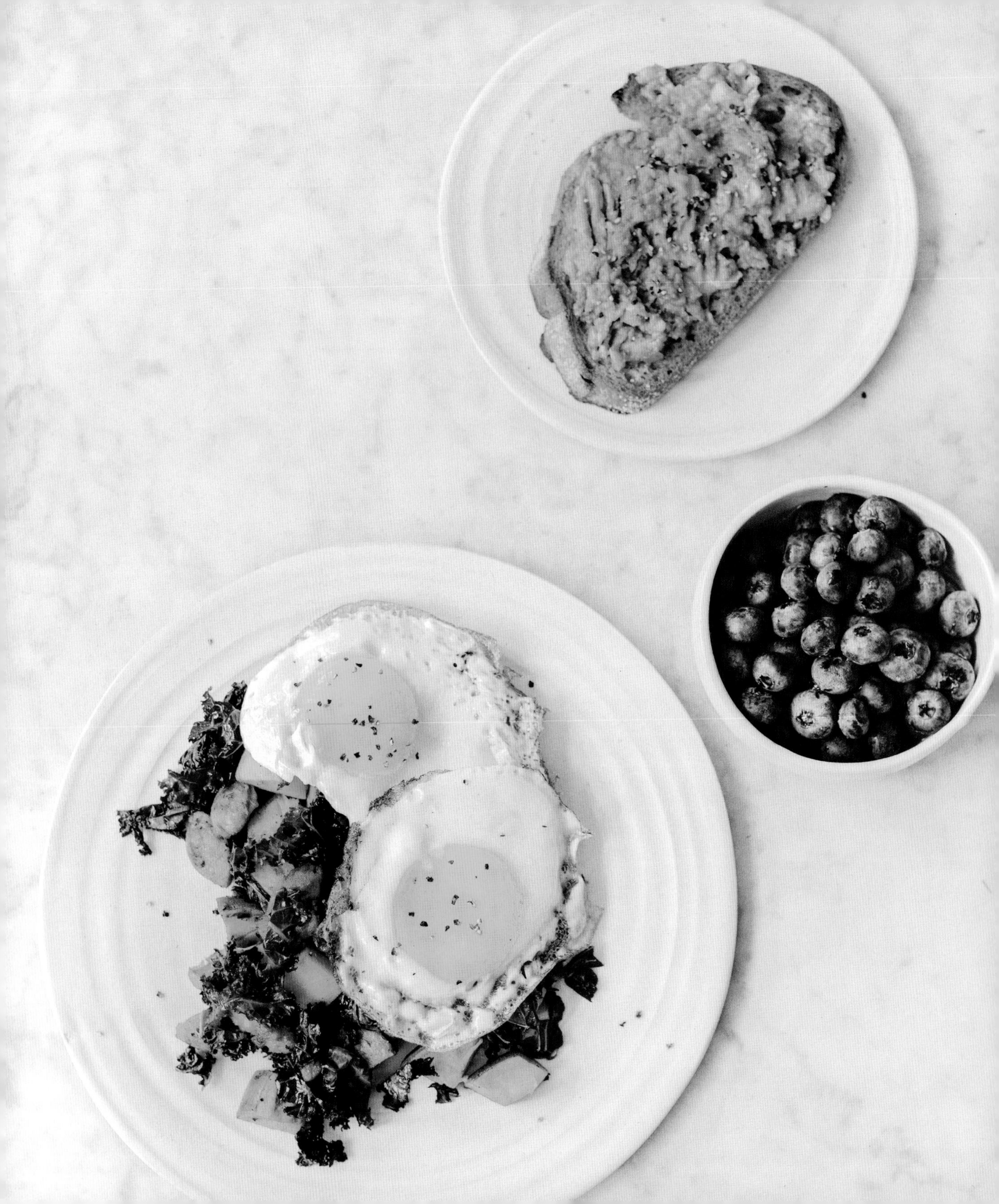

veggie-loaded all-american breakfast

The classic all-American breakfast has been taken up a few nutritional notches with some extra veggies and more fiber. This plate is perfect for slower mornings when there's a bit more time to make a tasty and hearty—but also blood sugar–balancing—breakfast. The fiber and protein in this breakfast will keep your blood sugars steady as you head into your day!

high fiber | no added sugar | protein packed | yield: 1 serving

1 tsp cooking oil

½ small sweet potato, cut into small cubes

1 cup (67 g) coarsely chopped kale leaves, stems removed

2 oz (57 g) cooked low-sodium chicken sausage

2 large eggs

1 cup (125 g) fresh berries of choice

1 slice whole-grain bread

2 tbsp (22 g) mashed avocado

Heat the oil in a large skillet over medium heat. Tilt and turn the skillet to coat the bottom with the oil.

Add the sweet potato, kale, and chicken sausage to the skillet. Sauté them for 10 to 15 minutes, or until the sweet potato is tender and the kale is soft.

Transfer the veggie mixture to a plate and return the skillet to the heat. Crack the eggs into the skillet and prepare them as desired to your preferred doneness. Once they are cooked, serve them with the veggie mixture, berries, bread, and avocado.

STORAGE: Serve this breakfast immediately.

Estimated Nutrition Facts per Serving: 561 calories; 60 g carbs; 10 g fiber; 21 g sugar; 29 g protein; 25 g fat (6.5 g saturated fat); 820 mg sodium

grain-free coconut and almond waffles

Who doesn't love a stack of waffles in the morning? Grain-free flours have less of an impact on your blood sugars than traditional wheat or rice flours. And topping these waffles with lower-sugar syrup alternatives like nuts and almond butter make them the perfect low-sugar way to start your day!

gluten-free | high fiber | no added sugar | sodium aware | yield: 4 servings

⅔ cup (164 g) no-added-sugar applesauce

4 large eggs, beaten

2 tsp (10 ml) pure vanilla extract

2 tsp (10 ml) pure almond extract

1 cup (240 ml) milk of choice

½ cup (56 g) coconut flour

1 cup (96 g) almond flour

1 tbsp (12 g) baking powder

Cooking oil spray, as needed

Almond butter, sliced almonds, and toasted coconut (optional)

Preheat the waffle iron per the manufacturer's instructions.

Meanwhile, in a blender, combine the applesauce, eggs, vanilla, almond extract, milk, coconut flour, almond flour, and baking powder. Blend the ingredients for about 20 seconds, until the batter is smooth.

If your waffle iron does not have a nonstick surface, spray it lightly with cooking oil spray before proceeding.

Pour about 3 tablespoons (45 ml) of the batter into the waffle iron for each waffle (this amount also depends on the size of your waffle iron). Follow the instructions for your waffle iron to cook the waffles.

Carefully remove the waffle from the waffle iron and let each waffle cool on a wire rack. Top the waffles with the almond butter, sliced almonds, and toasted coconut (if using).

STORAGE: Make these waffles ahead of time and freeze them for an easy weekday breakfast.

TIP: These waffles can also be made into pancakes! Heat a large skillet over medium heat. Spray it with your preferred cooking spray, and let the cooking spray get hot before adding the batter to the skillet. Cook the pancakes for 4 to 5 minutes on each side, until they are golden brown.

Estimated Nutrition Facts per Serving without Optional Toppings: 354 calories; 24 g carbs; 9 g fiber; 10 g sugar; 16 g protein; 22 g fat (5 g saturated fat); 141 mg sodium

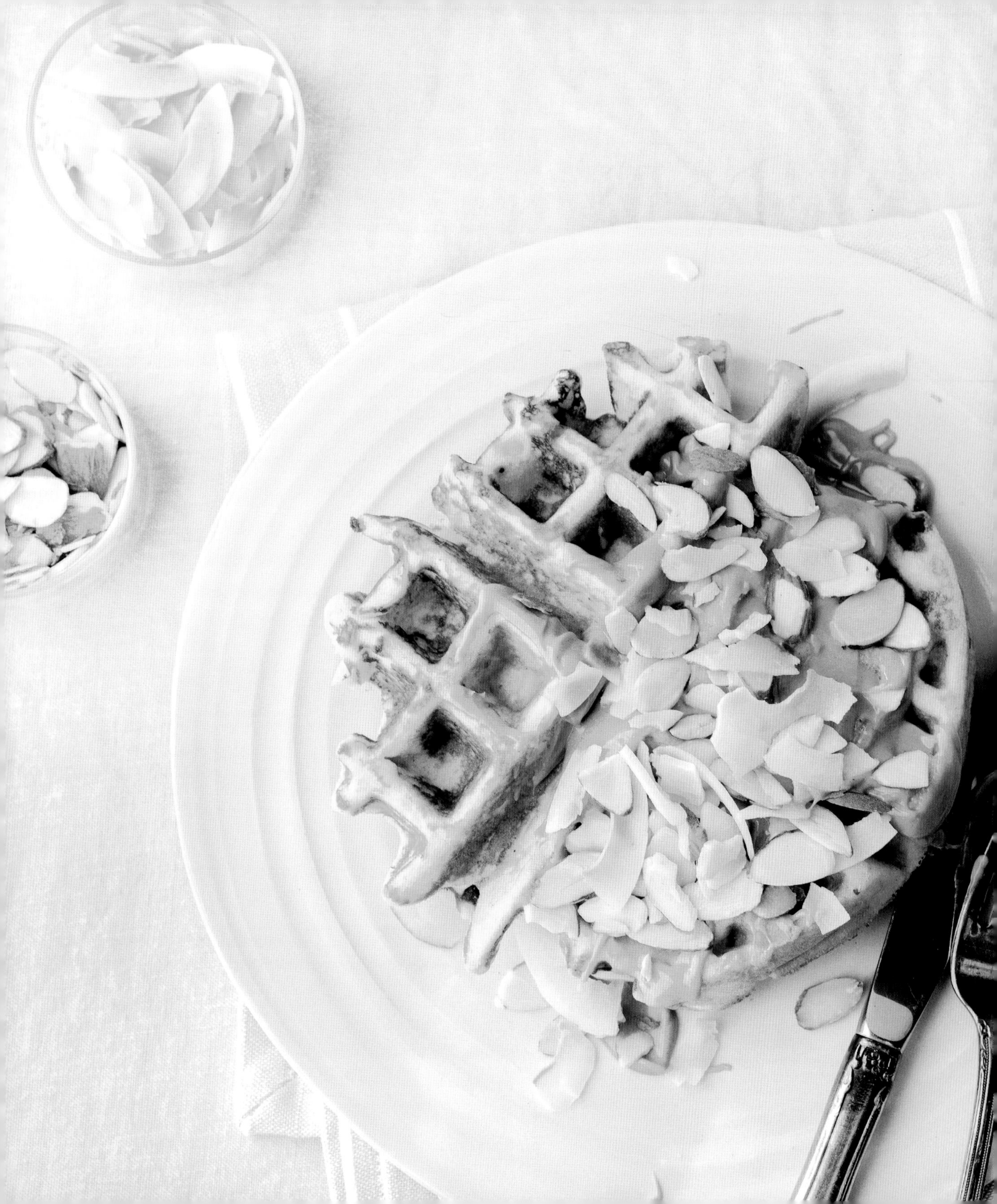

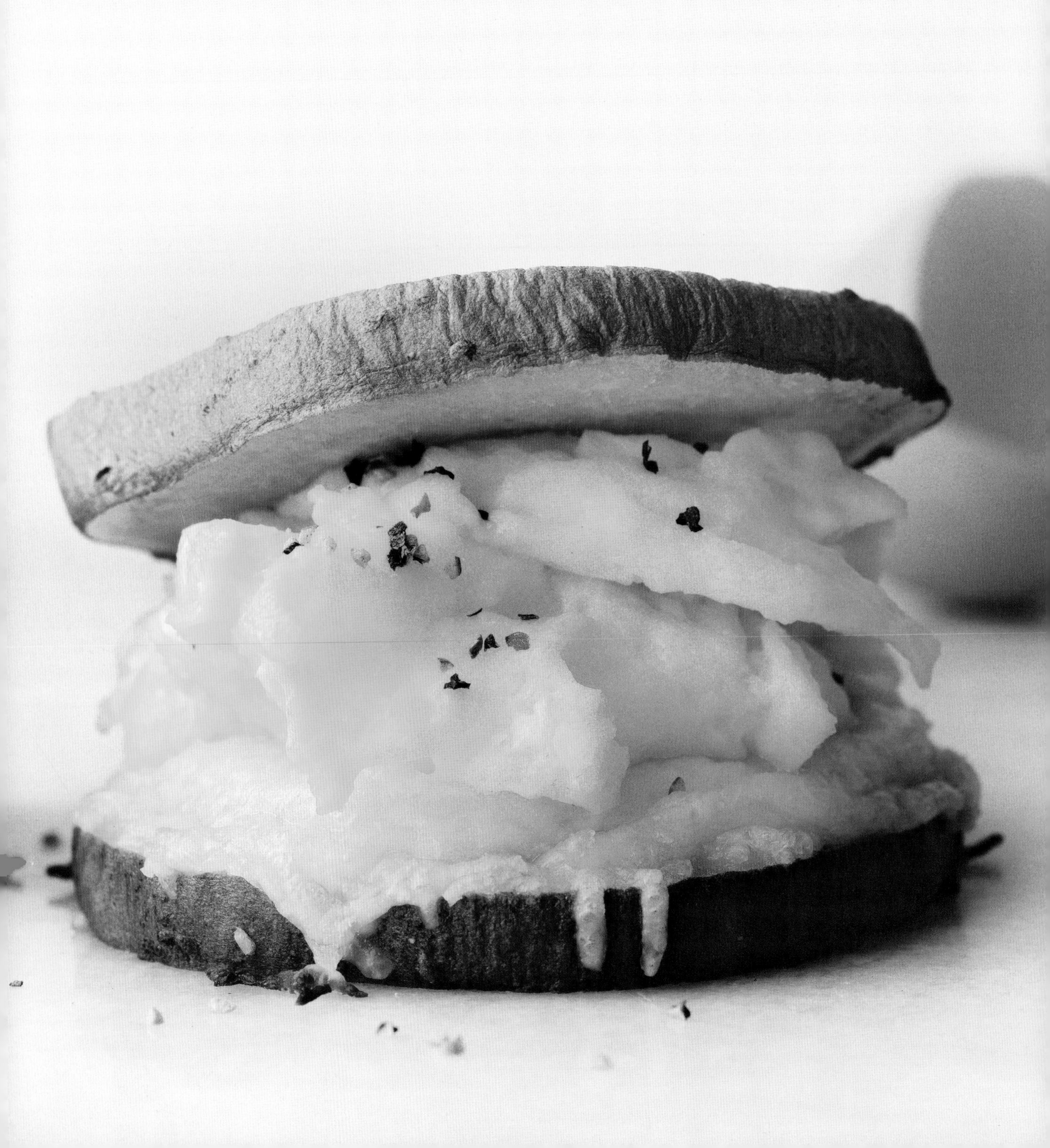

easy sweet potato and egg sandwiches

This recipe uses one of my favorite food trends from the past several years: sweet potato toast! Sweet potatoes are packed with vitamins, minerals, and fiber. When we swap traditional bread for sweet potato slices, we're lowering the carbohydrate content and upping the flavor and fiber content! Serve this sandwich up with a side of your favorite fruit and plant-based fat, like some avocado slices, for a complete and balanced meal.

gluten-free | no added sugar | yield: 2 servings

1 large sweet potato, sliced into 4 (¼-inch [6-mm]-thick) rounds

2 oz (57 g) shredded mozzarella cheese

Cooking oil spray, as needed

2 large eggs

Preheat the oven to broil. Line a large baking sheet with parchment paper.

Arrange the sweet potato rounds evenly on the prepared baking sheet. Broil the sweet potatoes for 4 to 6 minutes, until they are beginning to brown. Make sure to keep an eye on them so they don't burn.

Remove the sweet potatoes from the oven and add 1 ounce (28 g) of mozzarella cheese per sweet potato round to two of the rounds. Remove the plain sweet potato rounds from the baking sheet, and return the baking sheet with the cheese-topped sweet potatoes to the oven. Broil the rounds for 1 to 2 minutes, until the cheese begins to brown.

Remove the baking sheet from the oven and set it aside with the other sweet potato rounds.

Heat a medium skillet over medium heat. Spray it with the cooking oil spray and add the eggs. Scramble the eggs to your preferred doneness.

Top the cheesy sweet potato rounds with some of the scrambled eggs and the remaining sweet potato rounds. Slice the sandwiches and serve them.

STORAGE: Eat these sandwiches immediately.

Estimated Nutrition Facts per Serving: 222 calories; 20 g carbs; 3 g fiber; 4 g sugar; 15 g protein; 9 g fat (4 g saturated fat); 297 mg sodium

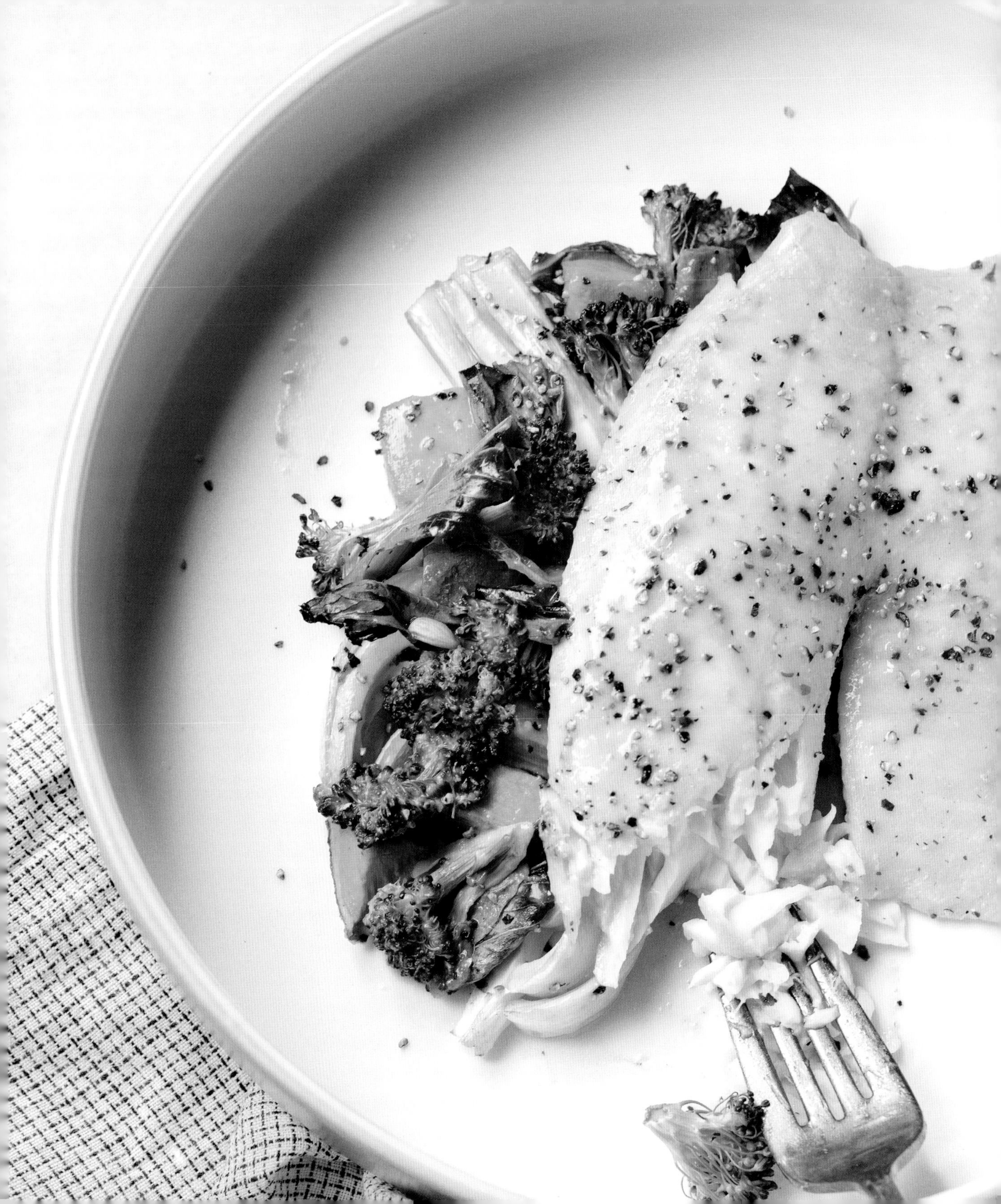

quick and delicious entrées

EASY RECIPES PERFECT FOR ANY NIGHT OF THE WEEK

Even when we do have time to cook dinner on a weeknight, no one wants to be stuck in the kitchen hovering over the stove for an hour. I am all about short and easy recipes that can feed my whole family and help me balance my blood sugars.

When it comes to choosing entrées that I know will help make my post-meal blood sugars more stable, there are a few questions I like to ask:

- **Does it have a quality protein source?** Good-quality protein—things like fish, chicken, lean red meat, tofu, beans, and so on—helps slow down digestion, which means blood sugars won't rise as quickly.
- **Is there at least 1 cup (240 g) of veggies in each serving?** If not, I make sure to pair it with another veggie recipe. Many of the recipes in this chapter pair perfectly with the recipes in the Flavorful Veggies chapter (page 97). A diet high in vegetables and fiber has been shown to be associated with fewer complications from diabetes, such as heart disease.
- **What types of sauces are used?** A really high-fat sauce can make post-meal blood sugars difficult to predict, as it drastically slows down how fast your body absorbs the carbohydrates. I recommend sauces that are low to moderate in fat and made primarily with plant-based fats like oils, nuts, seeds, and avocados.
- **Is it easy to prepare?** Again, if a certain recipe or dish adds stress to my plate, I tend to stay away from it. No one needs extra stress about food in their life.
- **Do I enjoy it?** This should be a given, but many people still try to force themselves to eat bland and boring dishes because that's what they think diabetes means. Hopefully by now you recognize that you can have delicious food, even with diabetes!

These recipes will have you in and out of the kitchen and on to more important things, like spending time with your family or catching up with friends, all while making sure your blood sugars stay balanced and steady after dinner.

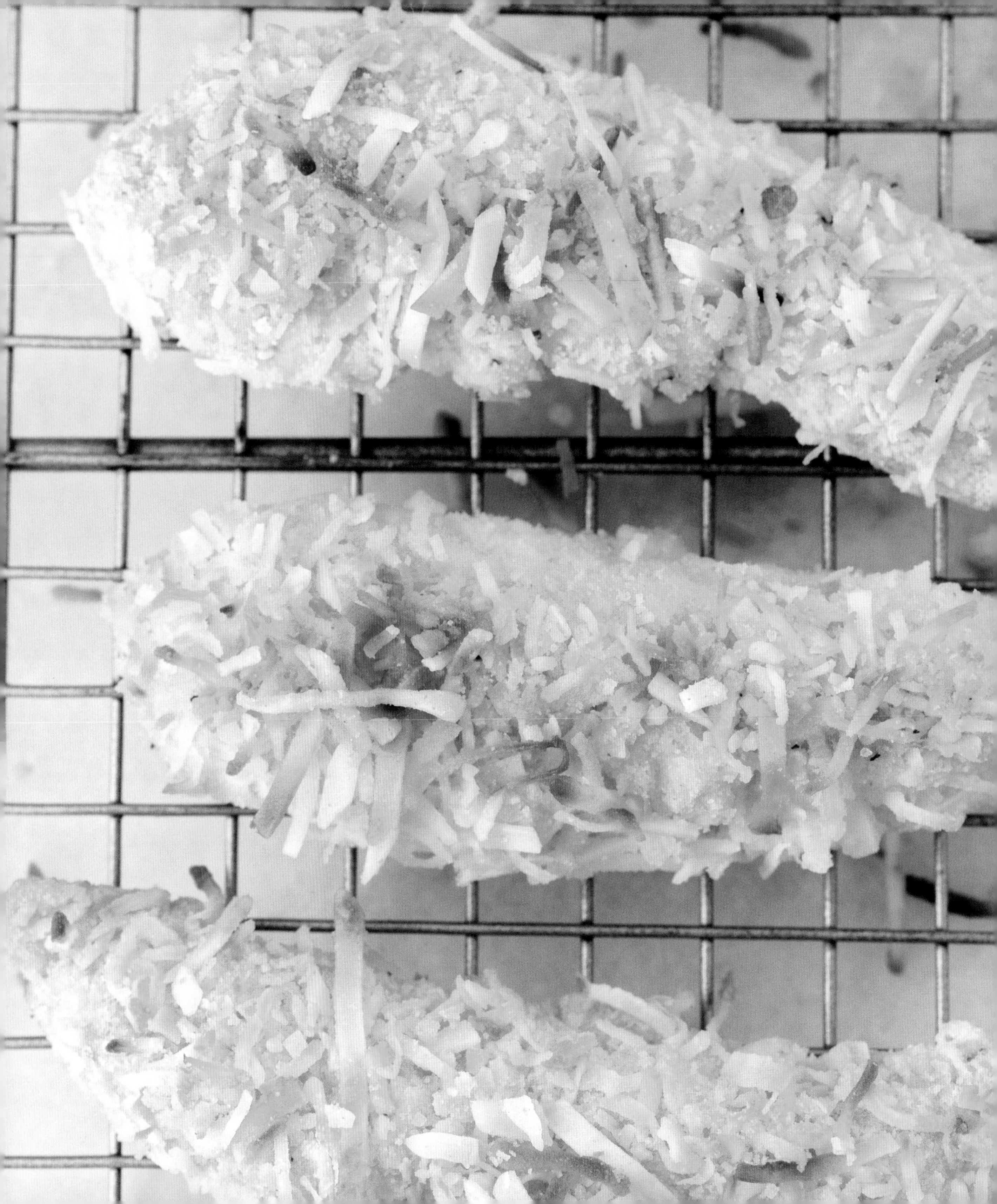

coconut-crusted chicken tenders

These chicken tenders go great in lunchboxes, on top of salads, or as a main dish served with veggies, like my Classic Oven-Roasted Carrots (page 100). Coconut flour is more blood sugar–friendly and offers a much tastier option than traditional flour for breading chicken and fish.

gluten-free | low carb | no added sugar | protein packed | yield: 6 servings

2 large eggs

1 cup (80 g) unsweetened coconut flakes

¼ cup (28 g) coconut flour

½ tsp garlic powder

½ tsp sea salt

2 lbs (907 g) boneless, skinless chicken breast tenders

Preheat the oven to 400°F (204°C). Line a large baking sheet with parchment paper.

Crack the eggs into a wide, shallow bowl and whisk them thoroughly to make an egg wash. Set the bowl aside.

In a medium bowl, combine the coconut flakes, coconut flour, garlic powder, and salt. Gently stir the ingredients to combine them. Spread the breading mixture out on a large plate.

Carefully dip each chicken tender in the egg wash, shaking off any excess egg wash. Dip the chicken tender in the coconut breading mixture, making sure to coat all sides. Place each coated chicken tender on the prepared baking sheet, being sure to space them at least 1 inch (2.5 cm) apart.

Bake the chicken tenders for 15 to 20 minutes, or until they are golden brown on the outside and no pink remains on the inside when you cut into them. Serve them immediately.

STORAGE: These are best eaten right away or frozen for a quick and easy weeknight meal. To freeze, let the chicken tenders cool to room temperature and then place the baking sheet directly in the freezer. After 1 to 2 hours, remove the chicken tenders from the baking sheet and place them in a large, freezer-safe bag. Store the tenders in the freezer for up to 3 months.

Estimated Nutrition Facts per Serving: 264 calories; 6 g carbs; 3 g fiber; <1 g sugar; 38 g protein; 9 g fat (6 g saturated fat); 326 mg sodium

30-minute garlic lamb lollipops

A 3-ounce (85-g) serving of lamb contains 3 grams of "good" fats, and 57 percent of the fat in lean cuts of lamb is monounsaturated, the same kind of fat found in olive oil! Lamb is a flavorful, nutrient-rich food and an excellent source of protein, zinc, selenium, riboflavin, niacin, vitamin B_{12}, and vitamin B_6. It's also super easy to prepare with the right cuts. This recipe is perfect for special occasions!

gluten-free | low carb | no added sugar | yield: 4 servings

2 tbsp (18 g) minced garlic

¼ cup (60 ml) avocado or olive oil

2 tbsp (30 ml) red wine vinegar

1 tbsp (3 g) Italian seasoning

½ tsp sea salt

¼ tsp black pepper

12 to 16 oz (340 to 454 g) lamb rib chops

1 tbsp (15 ml) avocado or grapeseed oil

Minced fresh rosemary, thyme, or basil, as needed

In a small bowl, combine the garlic, avocado oil, vinegar, Italian seasoning, salt, and black pepper. Whisk to mix the ingredients.

Place the lamb rib chops in an airtight container, like a plastic bag or glass storage container. Pour the marinade over the lamb rib chops and let them marinate at room temperature for 10 to 15 minutes.

Heat the avocado or grapeseed oil in a large cast-iron skillet over medium-high heat. Gently add the lamb rib chops to the skillet and cook them for 4 minutes. Flip the lamb and cook the meat for another 4 minutes, until it is brown on both sides.

Remove the lamb rib chops from the skillet, and let them rest for 10 minutes before serving. Garnish them with the herbs and serve.

STORAGE: Store the lamb lollipops in a sealed container in the refrigerator for up to 3 days.

Estimated Nutrition Facts per Serving: 568 calories; 2 g carbs; 0 g fiber; 0 g sugar; 19 g protein; 54.5 g fat (18 g saturated fat); 361 mg sodium

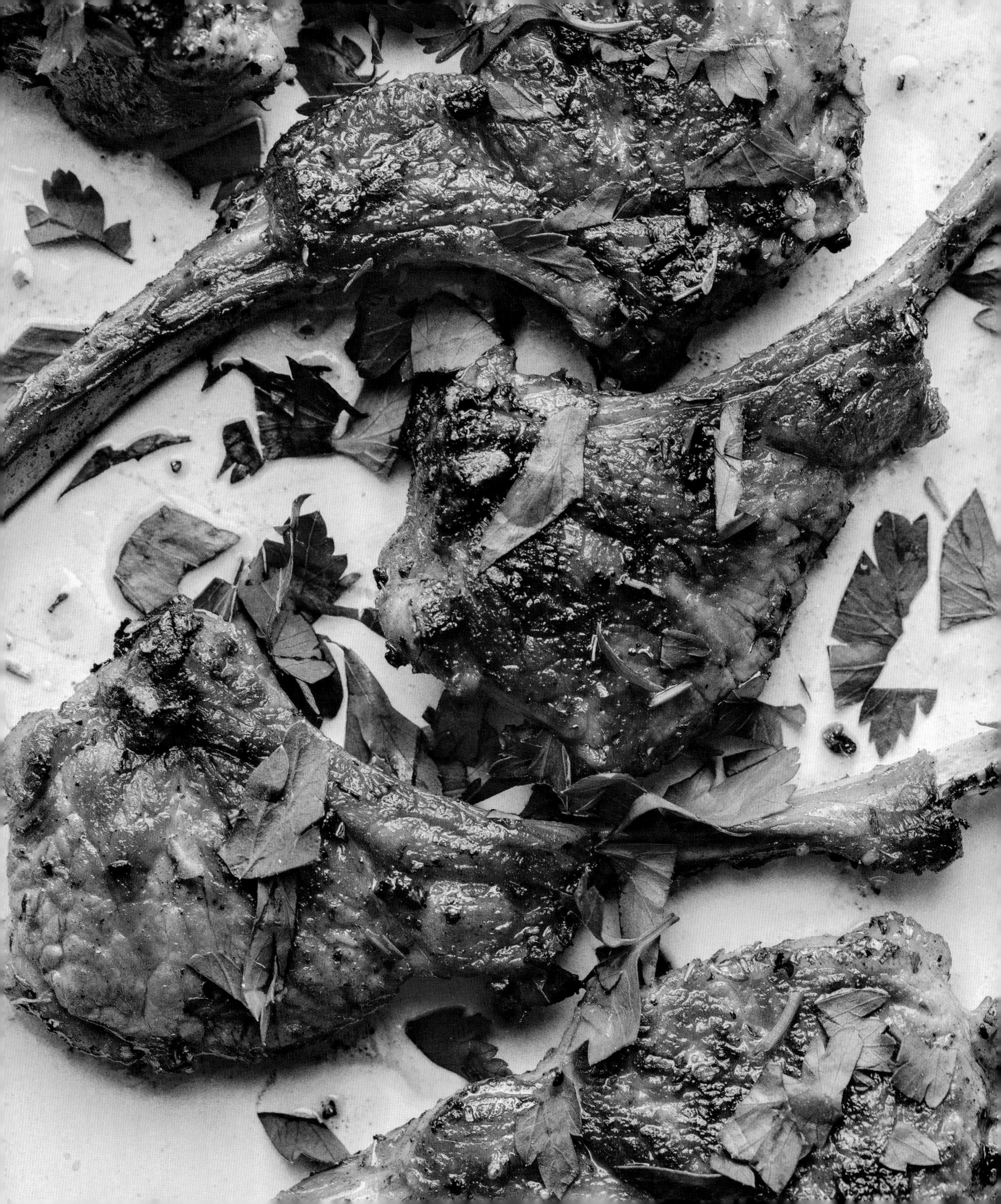

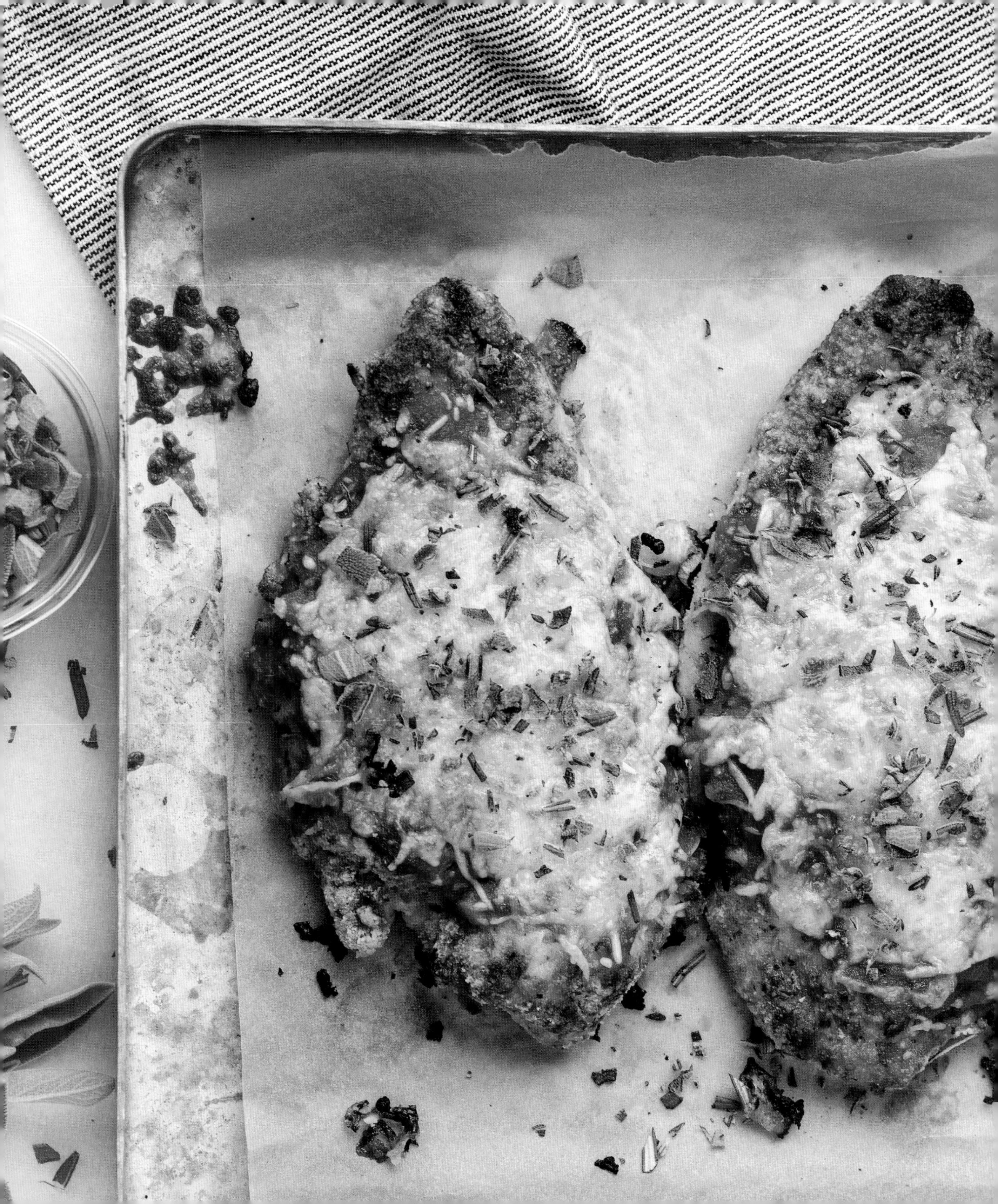

grain-free parmesan chicken

Traditional Parmesan chicken often uses refined breadcrumbs, but here we've replaced those with a much more blood sugar–friendly alternative: almond flour. Almond flour reduces the carbohydrate content of the dish and also adds plant-based fats for an equally nutritious and delicious meal!

gluten-free | high fiber | low carb | no added sugar | protein packed | yield: 4 servings

1½ cups (144 g) almond flour

½ cup (50 g) grated Parmesan cheese

1 tbsp (3 g) Italian seasoning

1 tsp garlic powder

½ tsp black pepper

2 large eggs

4 (6-oz [170-g], ½-inch [13-mm]-thick) boneless, skinless chicken breasts

½ cup (120 ml) no-added-sugar marinara sauce

½ cup (56 g) shredded mozzarella cheese

2 tbsp (8 g) minced fresh herbs of choice (optional)

Preheat the oven to 375°F (191°C). Line a large, rimmed baking sheet with parchment paper.

In a shallow dish, mix together the almond flour, Parmesan cheese, Italian seasoning, garlic powder, and black pepper. In another shallow dish, whisk the eggs. Dip a chicken breast into the egg wash, then gently shake off any extra egg. Dip the chicken breast into the almond flour mixture, coating it well. Place the chicken breast on the prepared baking sheet. Repeat this process with the remaining chicken breasts.

Bake the chicken for 15 to 20 minutes, or until the meat is no longer pink in the center.

Remove the chicken from the oven and flip each breast. Top each breast with 2 tablespoons (30 ml) of marinara sauce and 2 tablespoons (14 g) of mozzarella cheese.

Increase the oven temperature to broil and place the chicken back in the oven. Broil it until the cheese is melted and just starting to brown. Carefully remove the chicken from the oven, top it with the herbs (if using), and let it rest for about 10 minutes before serving.

STORAGE: Store the Parmesan chicken in a sealed container in the refrigerator for up to 3 days.

Estimated Nutrition Facts per Serving: 572 calories; 13 g carbs; 5 g fiber; 4 g sugar; 60 g protein; 32 g fat (7 g saturated fat); 560 mg sodium

meatless monday spinach lasagna

Who says lasagna can't be a nutrient-dense meal? With some small adjustments, we've packed this longtime favorite with 13 grams of fiber and 24 grams of protein to keep your blood sugars balanced and your taste buds satisfied. You'll want to serve this Meatless Monday Spinach Lasagna any day of the week!

gluten-free | high fiber | no added sugar | protein packed | yield: 4 servings

Cooking oil spray, as needed

2 large zucchini, quartered

1 cup (246 g) low-fat ricotta cheese (see Tips)

¼ cup (6 g) fresh basil leaves

2 tsp (2 g) dried oregano

Black pepper, as needed

2 cups (60 g) baby spinach

2 (15-oz [425-g]) cans no-salt-added tomato sauce

8 oz (227 g) no-boil chickpea lasagna noodles (see Tips)

½ cup (56 g) low-fat shredded mozzarella cheese

Preheat the oven to 375°F (191°C).

Spray a large skillet with the cooking oil spray. Heat the skillet over medium heat. Add the zucchini and sauté them for 7 to 10 minutes, or until they are tender.

Meanwhile, combine the ricotta, basil, oregano, black pepper, and spinach in a food processor and process until the mixture is combined. Alternatively, combine the ingredients in a medium bowl and stir to mix them together.

Coat the bottom of a 9 x 13–inch (23 x 32.5–cm) baking dish with a thin layer of the tomato sauce to ensure the bottom pasta layer doesn't burn. Add the first layer of lasagna noodles followed by one-fourth of the ricotta mixture and one-fourth of the cooked zucchini. Continue to layer the tomato sauce, noodles, ricotta, and zucchini. Finish the lasagna with a top layer of noodles, tomato sauce, and the mozzarella cheese.

Cover the lasagna with foil and bake it for 40 minutes. Remove the foil and bake it for 5 minutes, until the cheese is bubbly and slightly browned.

STORAGE: Store the lasagna in an airtight container in the refrigerator for up to 5 days.

Estimated Nutrition Facts per Serving: 384 calories; 51 g carbs; 13 g fiber; 16 g sugar; 24 g protein; 12 g fat (5 g saturated fat); 373 mg sodium

TIPS: For a higher-protein alternative, you can make tofu "ricotta" by blending together 6 to 8 ounces (170 to 227 g) of firm, drained tofu with ¼ cup (6 g) of fresh basil leaves, 2 teaspoons (2 g) of dried oregano, 1 tablespoon (15 ml) of fresh lemon juice, sea salt as needed, and black pepper as needed. Use this tofu "ricotta" as a 1:1 substitute for the ricotta cheese mixture.

Chickpea pasta is a high-protein, high-fiber alternative to typical boxed white-flour pasta.

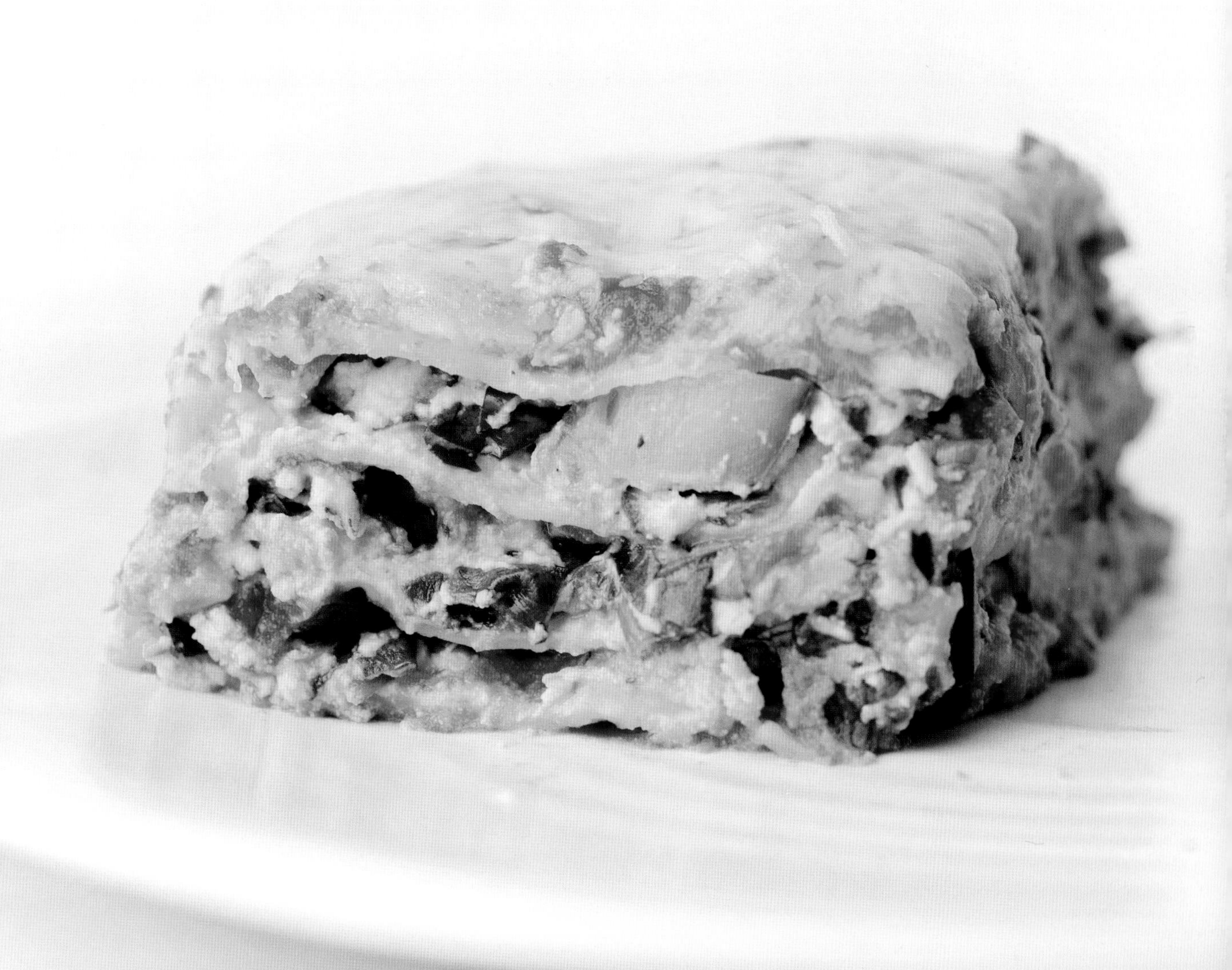

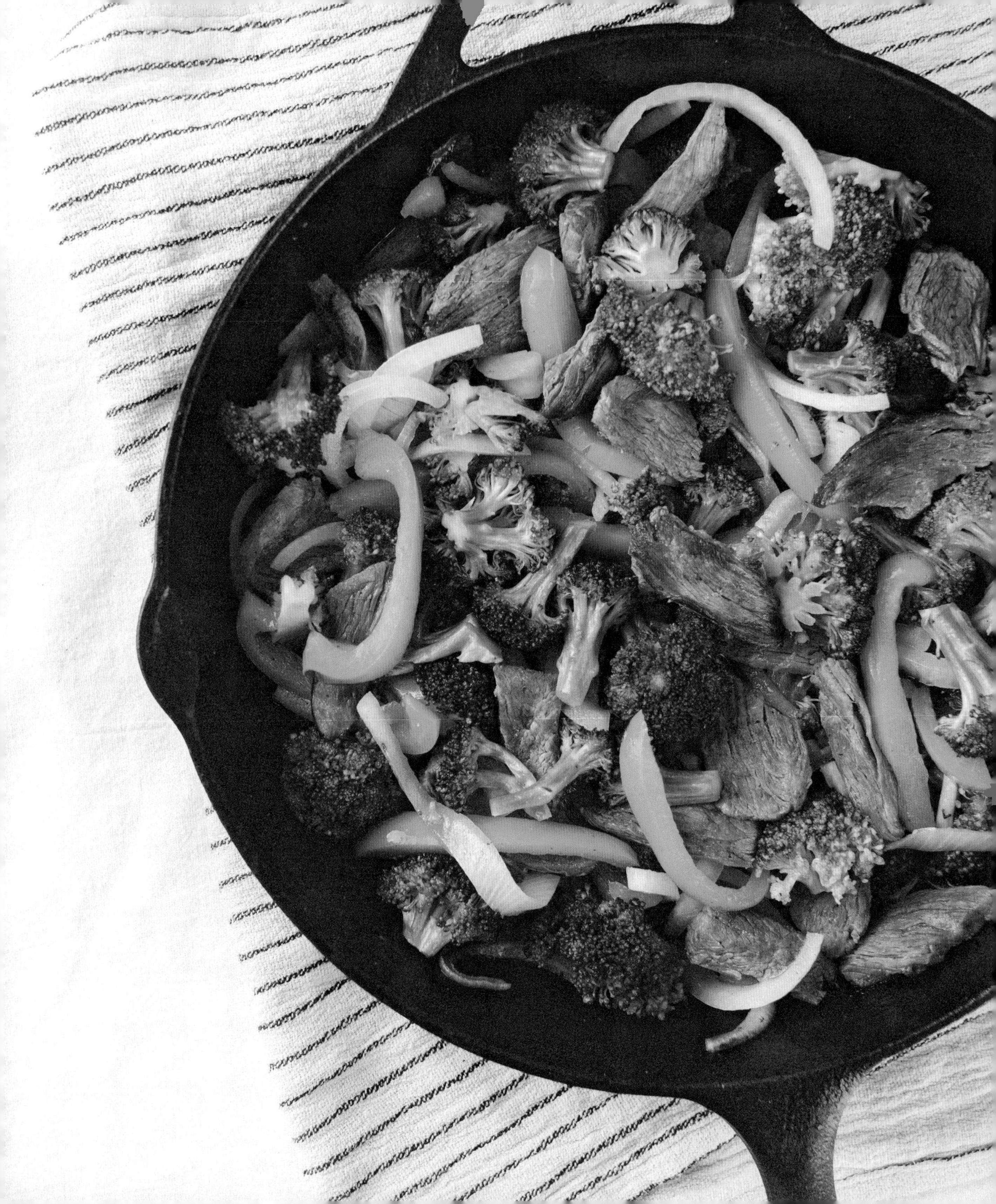

beef and broccoli stir-fry

Beef and broccoli is one of my favorite dishes to order at Asian restaurants, but the restaurant version is often packed with sugar. My homemade version is equally tasty but a lot lower in sugar and sodium. It's loaded with a few extra veggies, too, so you've got a complete meal ready to go!

gluten-free | protein packed | yield: 4 servings

1 cup (240 ml) low-sodium vegetable broth

1 tbsp (15 ml) low-sodium soy sauce or tamari

1½ tsp (5 g) garlic powder

1 tsp onion powder

¼ tsp ground ginger

¼ tsp black pepper

1 tbsp (15 ml) agave nectar

2 tsp (10 ml) rice wine vinegar

1 tbsp (9 g) tapioca flour or cornstarch

1 tbsp (15 ml) cooking oil of choice

1 lb (454 g) unseasoned skirt steak, cut into ½-inch (13-mm)-thick strips

1 medium white onion, thickly sliced

2 medium heads broccoli, cut into medium florets

2 medium orange bell peppers, thickly sliced

In a small bowl, combine the broth, soy sauce, garlic powder, onion powder, ginger, black pepper, agave nectar, vinegar, and tapioca flour. Mix the ingredients well with a fork and set the bowl aside.

Heat the cooking oil in a large skillet or wok over medium-high heat. Gently tilt the skillet to coat the bottom with the oil after it has become hot. Add the skirt steak to the skillet and cook it for 5 minutes, stirring frequently, making sure all sides of each strip of meat are browned.

Add the onion, broccoli, and bell peppers to the skillet. Cook the mixture for 5 to 6 minutes, stirring occasionally, until the vegetables have begun to soften.

Finally, add the broth mixture to the skillet and stir the beef and vegetables constantly for 2 to 3 minutes, or until the sauce begins to thicken. Remove the skillet from the heat and serve the stir-fry.

STORAGE: Store the stir-fry in a sealed container in the refrigerator for up to 3 days.

Estimated Nutrition Facts per Serving: 369 calories; 18 g carbs; 4 g fiber; 7 g sugar; 27 g protein; 21 g fat (8 g saturated fat); 258 mg sodium

easy spinach-artichoke enchilada casserole

Spinach and artichoke dip joins forces with enchiladas to create your new favorite casserole! Beans and artichokes pack this dish with fiber while the salsa and cheese pull everything together. With 14 grams of fiber and 19 grams of protein, your blood sugars will be nice and steady after dinner.

gluten-free | high fiber | no added sugar | yield: 4 servings

3 cups (500 g) frozen quartered artichoke hearts, thawed

1 medium onion, finely chopped

1 tsp dried oregano

1 clove garlic, minced

Black pepper, as needed

4 cups (120 g) baby spinach

1 (15-oz [425-g]) can white beans of choice, drained and rinsed

8 (6-inch [15-cm]) corn tortillas

⅔ cup (75 g) shredded Mexican cheese blend

¾ cup (180 ml) salsa verde

Salsa, sliced avocado, fresh lime juice, and finely chopped cilantro (optional)

Preheat the oven to 400°F (204°C).

Heat a large skillet over medium heat. Add the artichoke hearts, onion, oregano, garlic, and black pepper. Cook the mixture for 7 to 10 minutes, or until the onion is translucent and the artichoke hearts are browned. During the final minute of cooking, add the spinach and beans and cook until the spinach has wilted.

In a 9 x 13–inch (23 x 32.5–cm) baking dish, layer 2 tortillas, 2 to 3 tablespoons (14 to 21 g) of the Mexican cheese blend, 3 to 4 tablespoons (45 to 60 ml) of the salsa verde, and one-fourth of the bean and veggie mixture. Repeat this order until you've used all your ingredients.

Cover the casserole with foil or an oven-safe lid and bake it for 20 minutes, or until the cheese has melted. Serve the casserole with the salsa, avocado, lime juice, and cilantro (if using).

STORAGE: Store the casserole in a sealed container in the refrigerator for up to 5 days.

Estimated Nutrition Facts per Serving: 368 calories; 59 g carbs; 14 g fiber; 3 g sugar; 19 g protein; 7 g fat (6 g saturated fat); 546 mg sodium

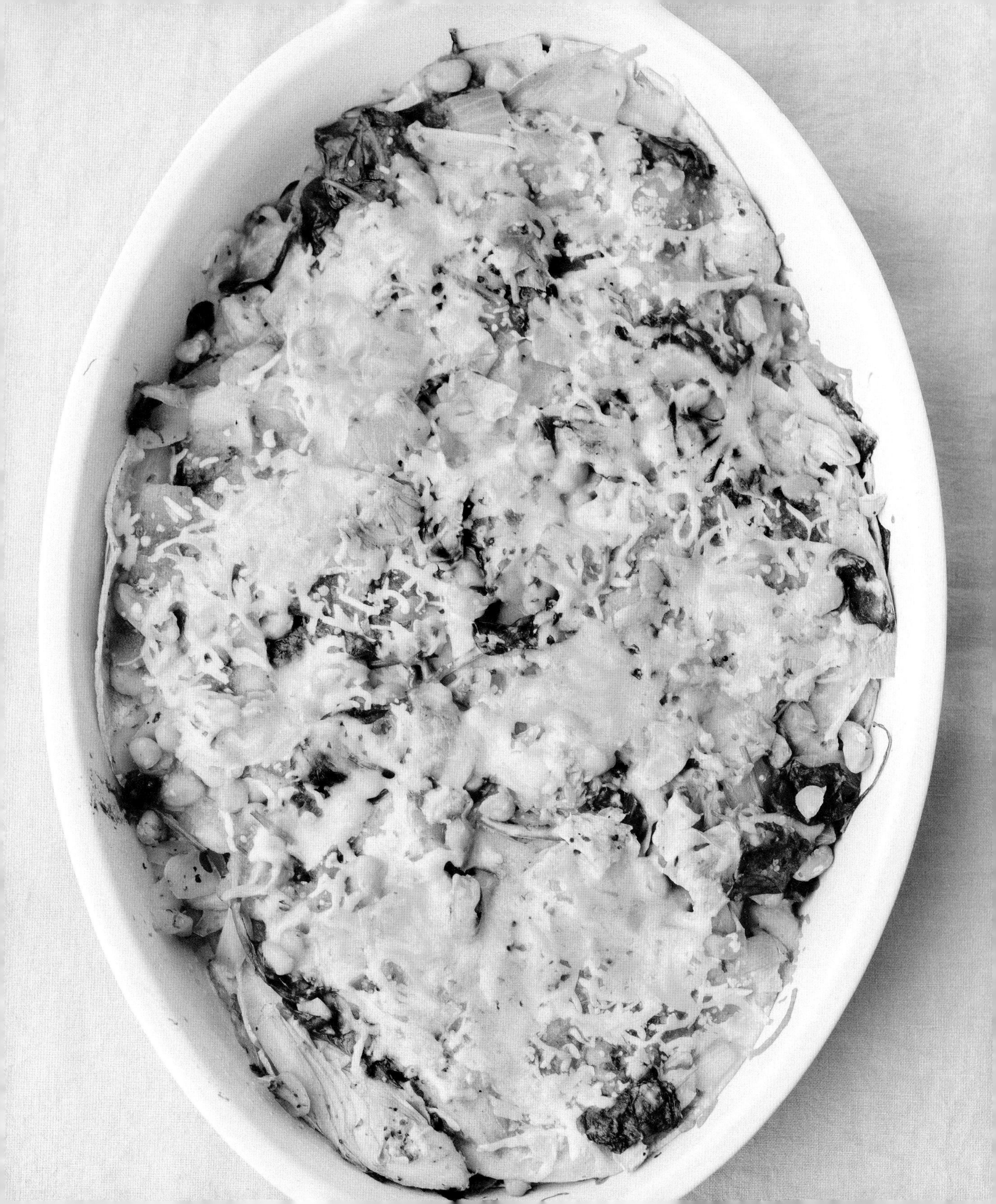

sheet pan tilapia two ways

Get your dinner from oven to table in less than 30 minutes with this nutritious and versatile meal! Tilapia is a quick-cooking, low-fat, and high-protein staple to pair with your favorite veggies and starch. It's a quality source of protein that is perfect for balancing blood sugars. Choose the Miso-Glazed Tilapia or the Lemon, Oregano, and Dill Tilapia. Both options boost the fiber of your dinner, which, like the protein, will help you feel fuller longer and prevent any post-meal blood sugar spikes.

miso-glazed tilapia: gluten-free | high fiber | protein packed
lemon, oregano, and dill tilapia: gluten-free | no added sugar | protein packed | sodium aware
yield: 4 servings

miso-glazed tilapia

1½ tbsp (26 g) miso of choice

¼ cup (60 ml) water

1 tsp ground ginger

½ tsp garlic powder

1 tsp sesame oil

1 tsp honey

1 tsp apple cider vinegar

2 cups (350 g) broccoli florets, cut into 1-inch (2.5-cm) pieces

2 large sweet potatoes, cut into 1-inch (2.5-cm) pieces

2 cups (140 g) coarsely chopped bok choy

1½ lbs (680 g) tilapia fillets

miso-glazed tilapia

Preheat the oven to 400°F (204°C).

In a medium bowl, whisk together the miso, water, ginger, garlic powder, sesame oil, honey, and vinegar. Set the bowl aside.

Spread the broccoli and sweet potatoes on a baking sheet and pour half the miso mixture over the vegetables. Bake the vegetables for 15 minutes. After 15 minutes, remove the baking sheet and make room on the baking sheet for the bok choy and tilapia, then place the bok choy and tilapia directly on the baking sheet. Drizzle the remaining miso mixture over everything. Bake the tilapia and vegetables for 10 minutes, until the sauce starts to bubble and the fish is cooked through.

Divide the tilapia and vegetables among four plates and serve.

Estimated Nutrition Facts per Serving: Miso-Glazed Tilapia: 338 calories; 34 g carbs; 6 g fiber; 9 g sugar; 39 g protein; 5 g fat (1 g saturated fat); 495 mg sodium

lemon, oregano, and dill tilapia

4 cups (700 g) broccoli florets, cut into 1-inch (2.5-cm) pieces

1 lb (454 g) yellow potatoes, cut into 1-inch (2.5-cm) pieces

1 tbsp (15 ml) olive oil

Juice of ½ medium lemon

2 tsp (2 g) dried oregano

2 tbsp (4 g) minced fresh dill or 2 tsp (2 g) dried dill

1½ lbs (680 g) tilapia fillets

½ medium lemon, thinly sliced

lemon, oregano, and dill tilapia

Preheat the oven to 400°F (204°C).

Place the broccoli and potatoes on a large baking tray.

In a small bowl, whisk together the oil, lemon juice, oregano, and dill. Pour half of the mixture over the vegetables. Bake the vegetables for 15 minutes.

After 15 minutes, remove the baking sheet and make room on it for the tilapia. Place the tilapia directly on the baking sheet. Cover the tilapia with the lemon slices. Drizzle the remaining marinade over everything. Bake the tilapia and vegetables for 10 minutes, until the fish is light brown on top and cooked through.

Divide the tilapia and vegetables among four plates and serve.

*See photo on page 36.

STORAGE: Store the tilapia and vegetables in a sealed container in the refrigerator for up to 2 days.

Lemon, Oregano, and Dill Tilapia: 312 calories; 27 g carbs; 4 g fiber; 2 g sugar; 39 g protein; 16 g fat (6 g saturated fat); 218 mg sodium

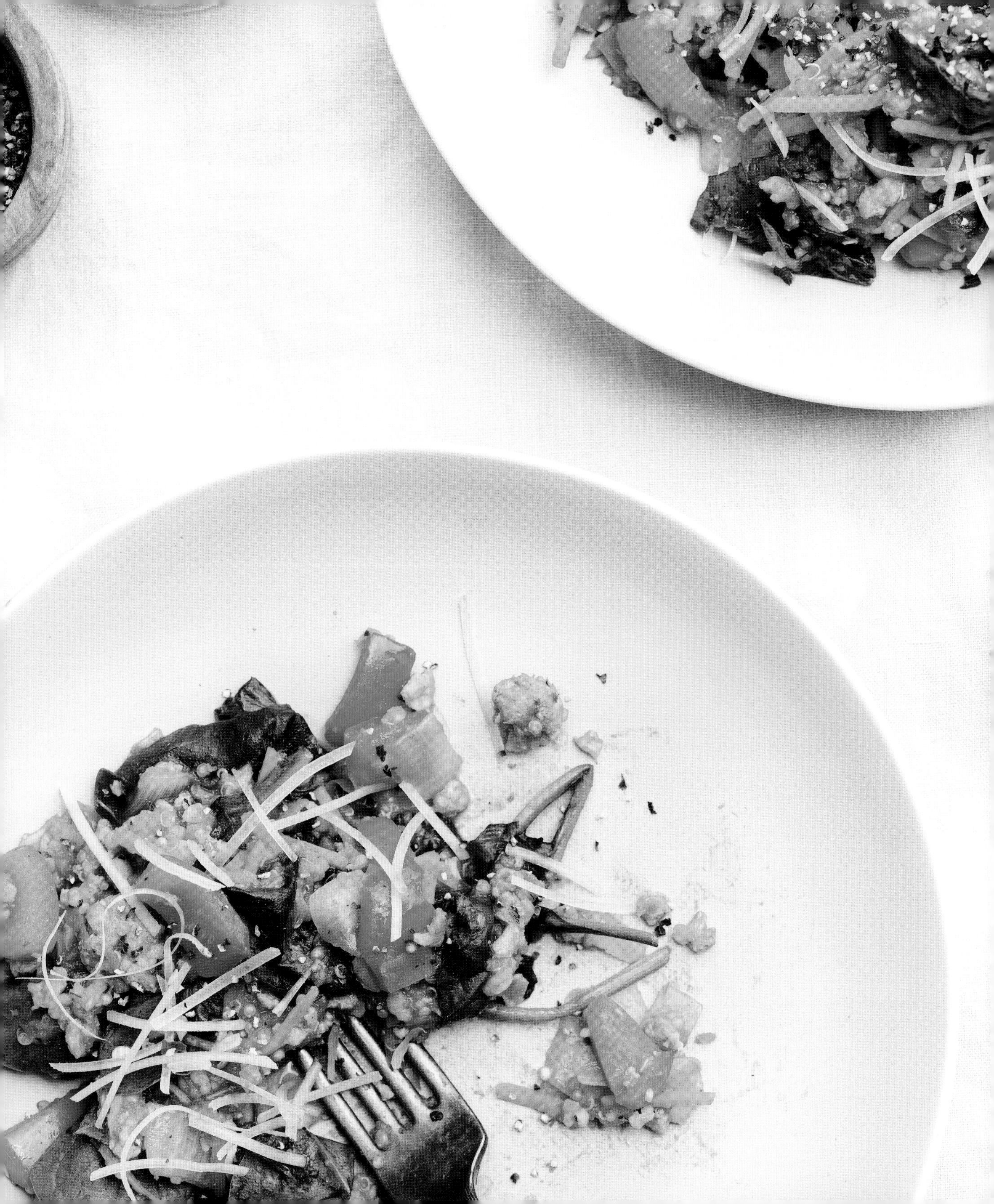

unstuffed bell peppers

One of my favorite meals to enjoy is stuffed bell peppers, but they typically take a long time to make and are loaded with large amounts of rice, meaning most versions are not very easy for people with diabetes to enjoy. This recipe boasts all the same flavors without a ton of labor, and we've replaced half of the rice with protein-packed quinoa. This is a dish everyone can enjoy!

gluten-free | high fiber | no added sugar | protein packed | yield: 5 servings

1 tbsp (15 ml) olive oil

1 medium yellow onion, coarsely chopped

4 medium red bell peppers, coarsely chopped

1 lb (454 g) ground turkey

10 oz (283 g) shredded carrots

1 cup (202 g) cooked brown rice

1 cup (185 g) cooked quinoa

3 cups (720 ml) no sugar-added marinara or seasoned tomato sauce (see Tips)

5 oz (142 g) baby spinach

Sea salt, as needed

Black pepper, as needed

½ cup (50 g) grated Parmesan cheese (optional)

Heat a large skillet over medium-high heat. Once the skillet is hot, add the oil and let it heat for 1 to 2 minutes.

Add the onion and bell peppers to the skillet and sauté them for 7 to 8 minutes, until the onion starts to become translucent.

Add the turkey and cook it for 8 to 10 minutes, until it is no longer pink and has browned slightly. Add the carrots, rice, and quinoa. Stir everything together.

Add the marinara, spinach, sea salt, and black pepper and cook the mixture for 2 to 3 minutes, stirring constantly, until the spinach is wilted. Stop stirring and cook the mixture for 3 to 5 minutes, until the sauce starts to bubble.

Remove the skillet from the heat and top the mixture with the Parmesan cheese (if using), then serve.

STORAGE: Store the Unstuffed Bell Peppers in an airtight container for up to 5 days in the refrigerator.

TIPS: To avoid a bland meal, be sure to buy a flavorful marinara sauce or a seasoned tomato sauce that uses garlic, Italian-inspired herbs, and so on.

To save even more time, buy your veggies prechopped and shredded. You can also cook the rice and quinoa yourself, but to save time on a busy weeknight, I recommend the microwavable pouches to make this recipe even easier and simpler.

Estimated Nutrition Facts per Serving: 409 calories; 43 g carbs; 10 g fiber; 16 g sugar; 22 g protein; 18 g fat (4 g saturated fat); 705 mg sodium

fiber-full chicken tostadas

These tostadas use my favorite taco seasoning blend to flavor the chicken. (I bet you have all the seasonings at home already—no need to buy premade taco seasoning!) By relying on toppings like beans, greens, and avocado slices, we've got 12 grams of fiber per serving to help keep blood sugars balanced. This makes a family-friendly weeknight meal.

gluten-free | high fiber | no sugar added | protein packed | yield: 4 servings

1 tbsp (9 g) chili powder

½ tbsp (5 g) onion powder

1 tbsp (9 g) paprika

1 tsp garlic powder

1 tsp ground cumin

1 tsp dried oregano

¼ tsp black pepper

¼ tsp sea salt

2 tbsp (30 ml) cooking oil of choice

1 lb (454 g) boneless, skinless chicken breast, cut into 1 to 1½-inch (2.5 to 3.8-cm) strips

8 corn tostada shells

1 (15.5-oz [439-g]) can low-sodium pinto beans, undrained

1 cup (30 g) baby arugula leaves, coarsely chopped

1 large avocado, peeled and sliced to the desired thickness

4 tbsp (32 g) crumbled queso fresco cheese

Jalapeño slices (optional)

Chopped onion (optional)

Diced tomatoes (optional)

In a small bowl, mix together the chili powder, onion powder, paprika, garlic powder, cumin, oregano, black pepper, and sea salt. Add the cooking oil and mix it with the seasonings to make a marinade.

Place the chicken strips in a large ziptop plastic bag, then add the marinade. Seal the bag and shake it to coat the chicken with the marinade. (If time permits, marinate the chicken for 30 to 60 minutes.)

Heat a large skillet over medium-high heat. Add the chicken strips and cook them for 4 to 5 minutes. Flip the chicken strips and cook them for 3 to 4 minutes, until they are cooked through and no longer pink. Set the skillet aside.

Line up the tostada shells on a serving tray. Place the pinto beans in a medium bowl and mash them to the desired consistency. Spread the beans on top of each tostada. Top each tostada with an equal amount of arugula, avocado slices, cheese, chicken and any desired additional toppings, then serve.

STORAGE: Serve the tostadas immediately.

TIP: Prep the chicken ahead of time to make assembly for dinner even quicker. Add extra toppings like jalapeño slices, chopped onion, or diced tomatoes to these tostadas if you like!

Estimated Nutrition Facts per Serving: 547 calories; 36 g carbs; 12 g fiber; 1 g sugar; 40 g protein; 27 g fat (8 g saturated fat); 738 mg sodium

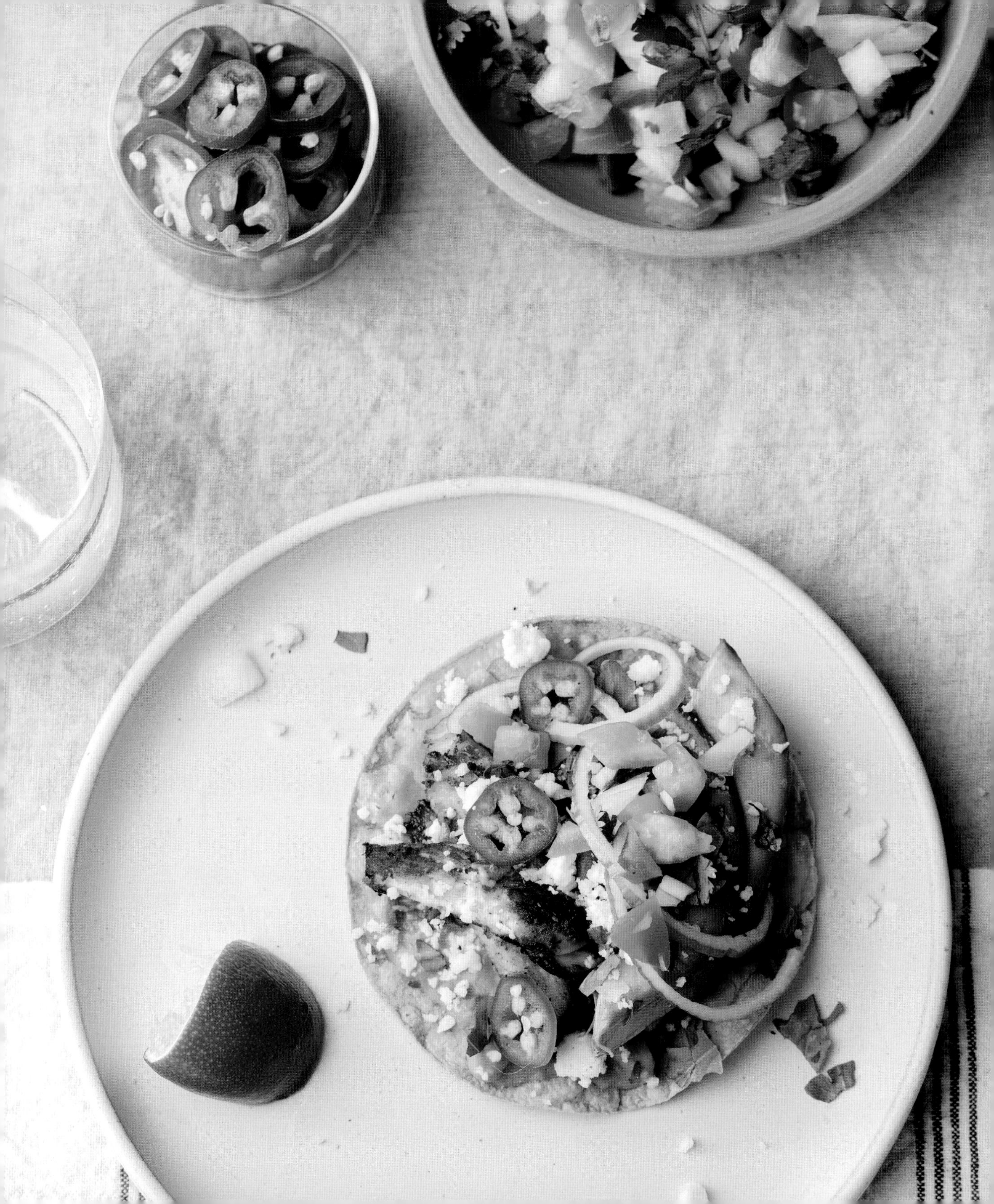

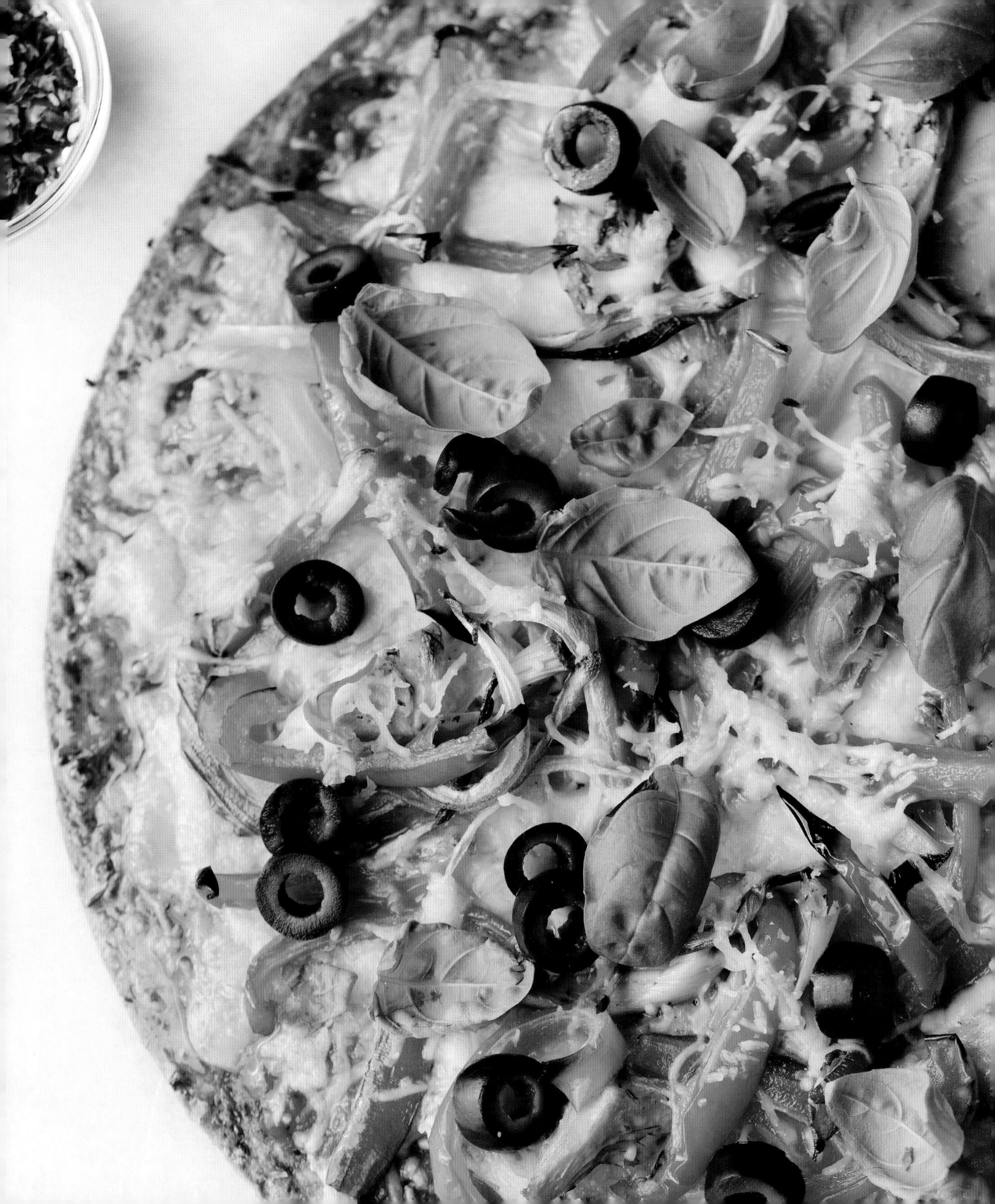

diabetes-friendly artichoke and basil pizza

A store-bought whole-grain crust becomes the perfect vehicle for a nutrient-packed pizza night! Your family's chefs can express their creativity with their favorite veggies, sauces, and spices as toppings. The following are just some of my high-fiber favorites. The added fiber can help prevent blood sugars from spiking after your meal.

protein packed | yield: 4 servings

Cooking oil spray, as needed

2 medium red bell peppers, thinly sliced

1 medium onion, thinly sliced

½ cup (85 g) canned quartered artichoke hearts, drained

1 (10-oz [283-g]) package whole-grain flatbread or pizza crust (see Tip)

½ cup (120 ml) tomato sauce

4 oz (113 g) shredded mozzarella cheese

¼ cup (32 g) sliced black olives

10 to 15 fresh basil leaves

Preheat the oven to 400°F (204°C).

Spray a large skillet with the cooking oil spray and set it over medium heat. Add the bell peppers, onion, and artichoke hearts, and cook the vegetables for about 5 minutes, until the onion is almost translucent.

Bake the pizza crust for 6 to 7 minutes. Remove the crust from the oven and layer on the tomato sauce, sautéed vegetables, and mozzarella cheese. Bake the pizza for 5 to 6 minutes, or until the cheese is melted.

Top the pizza with the olives and basil leaves and serve.

STORAGE: Store the pizza in a closed container in the refrigerator for up to 5 days.

TIP: While you will need to bake the crust according to the directions outlined here, be sure to read the crust's package on whether to bake the crust on a baking sheet or directly on the oven rack. Different types and brands of crust will have different requirements, so check the label on yours before proceeding.

Estimated Nutrition Facts per Serving: Nutrients will vary based on the pizza crust you choose.

quinoa and brown rice power bowl

Power through lunchtime with this delicious grain bowl. The fiber- and protein-packed ingredients will prevent the dreaded 3:00 p.m. slump, as cashews provide crunch and a dose of heart-healthy fats to keep you satiated until dinner. All three—fat, fiber, and protein—work together to make this power bowl a more blood sugar–friendly option than traditional grain-based bowls.

high fiber | no added sugar | yield: 4 servings

½ cup (95 g) uncooked brown rice

½ cup (85 g) uncooked quinoa

2 green onions, finely chopped, divided

2 tsp (6 g) ground ginger, divided

2 cloves garlic, finely chopped, divided

1 (14-oz [397-ml]) can light coconut milk (see Tips)

1 to 2 cups (240 to 480 ml) water (optional; see Tips)

4 cups (268 g) coarsely chopped kale

1 tbsp (15 ml) sesame oil

2 tbsp (30 ml) low-sodium soy sauce

2 tsp (6 g) ground coriander

Black pepper, as needed

¼ cup (28 g) raw cashews

Cooking oil spray, as needed

4 large eggs

½ cup (80 g) unsweetened dried cherries

1 small lime, quartered

Combine the rice, quinoa, 1 of the green onions, 1 teaspoon of the ginger, 1 clove of garlic, coconut milk, and water (if using) in a large pot and bring the mixture to a boil over high heat. Reduce the heat to low and simmer the mixture for about 20 minutes, or 22 to 23 minutes if using the optional water, until the liquid is absorbed.

In the meantime, combine the kale, oil, soy sauce, coriander, remaining green onion, remaining 1 teaspoon of ginger, and remaining clove of garlic in a large skillet over medium heat. Cook the mixture for 5 to 7 minutes, until the kale is bright green with crispy edges. After 3 to 5 minutes, add the black pepper and cashews to lightly toast the nuts. Remove the kale mixture from the skillet and set it aside while the brown rice and quinoa finish cooking.

Spray the skillet with the cooking oil spray and crack the eggs into the skillet. Cook the eggs over medium-high heat, until the yolks are cooked to your preference: about 2 minutes for medium yolks, or 3 to 4 minutes for well-set yolks.

Divide the brown rice and quinoa mixture among four bowls. Layer the kale mixture into each bowl, and top each serving with a fried egg, some dried cherries, and a quarter of the lime for a squeeze of lime juice.

STORAGE: Freeze the power bowls for up to 3 months or store them in the refrigerator in a sealed container for up to 5 days.

TIPS: Cooking the rice and quinoa in coconut milk infuses them with flavor and gives them a creamy texture.

Use the optional extra water if you prefer softer grains.

Estimated Nutrition Facts per Serving: 441 calories; 53 g carbs; 6 g fiber; 12 g sugar; 14 g protein; 19 g fat (8 g saturated fat); 254 mg sodium

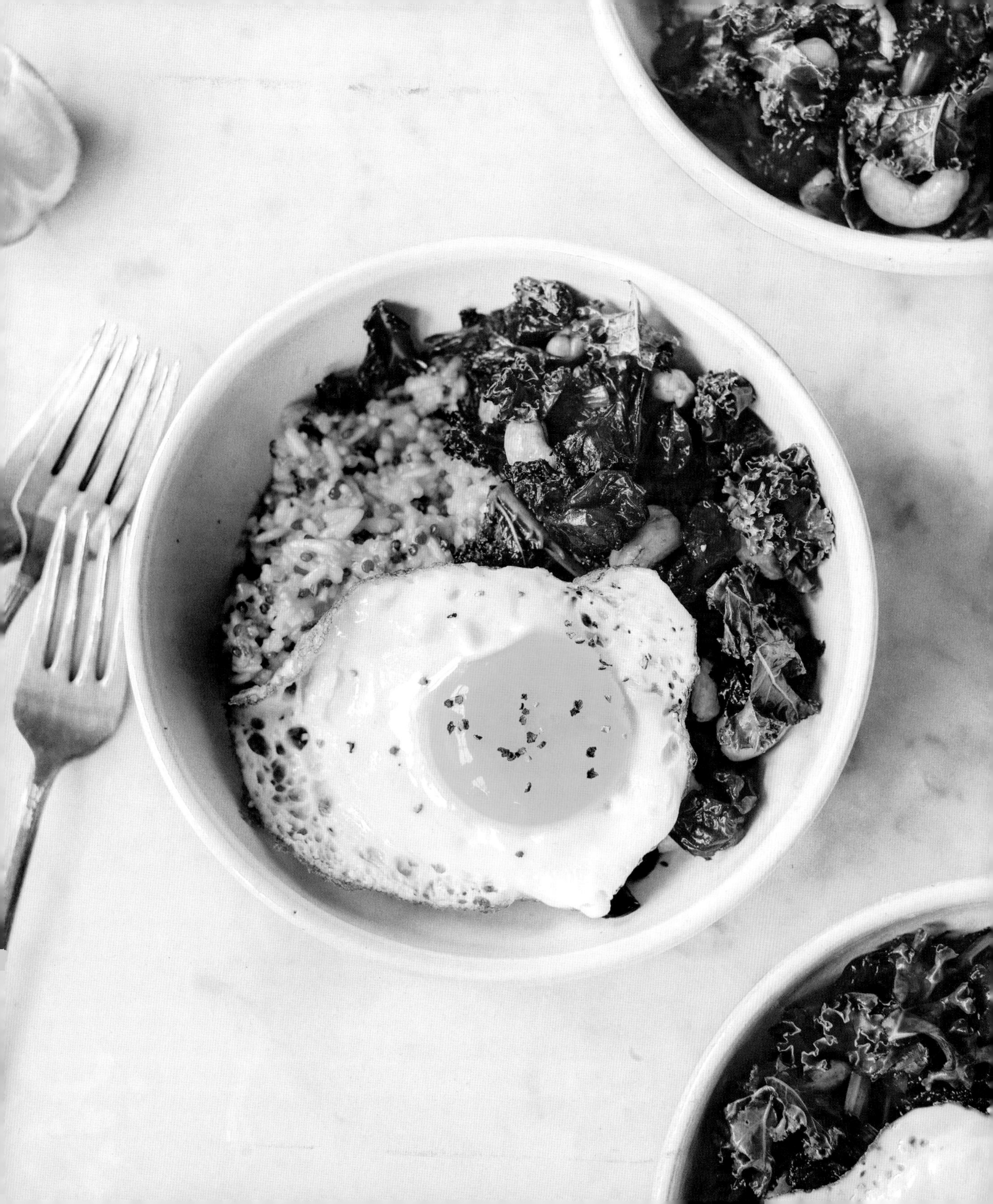

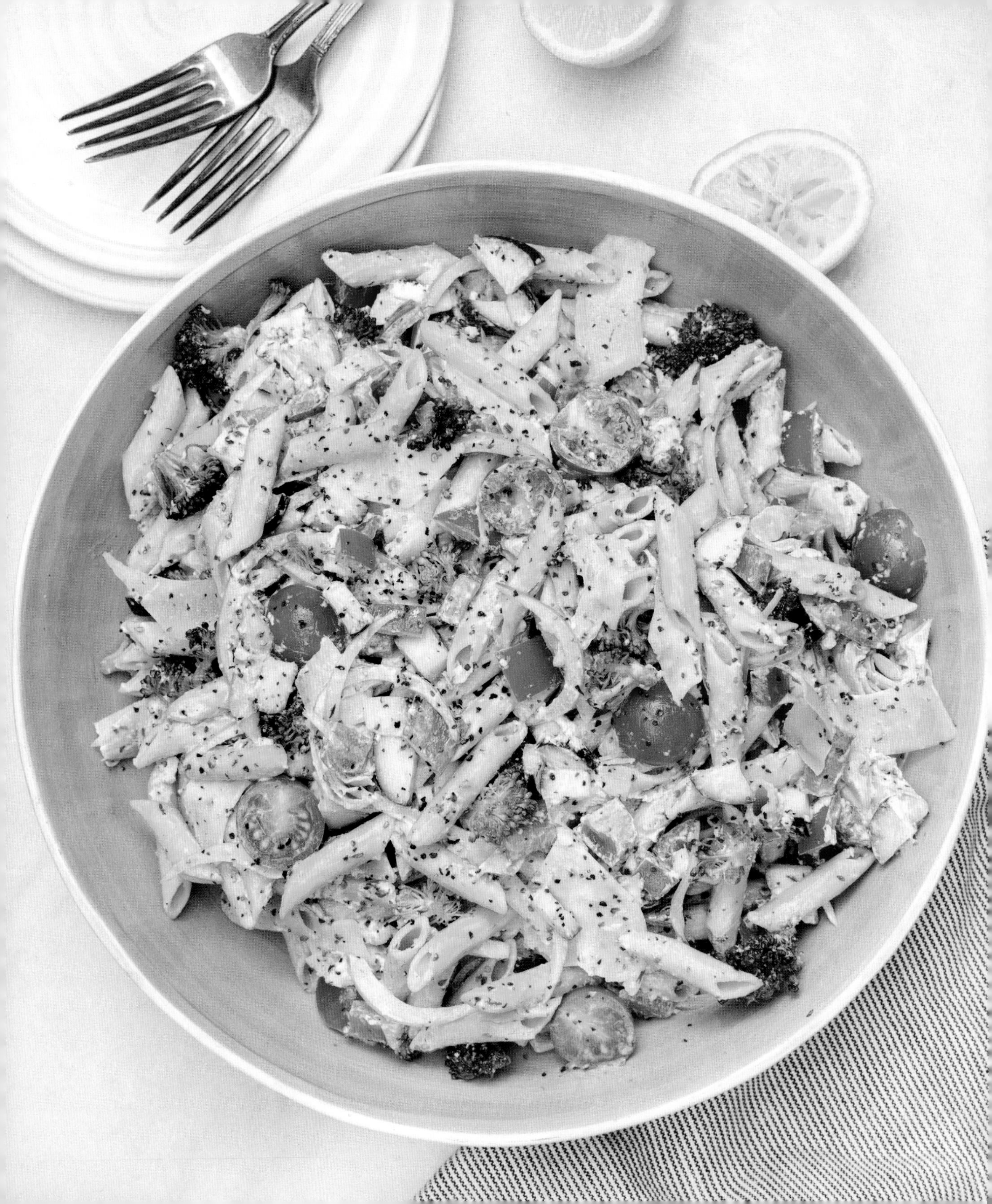

simple 15-minute meals

STRESS-FREE DINNER SOLUTIONS

Life is busy, and cooking a full meal each night isn't always an option. But unfortunately, many quick and easy dinner options aren't very good for balancing blood sugars. So what's a person living with diabetes to do? The recipes in this chapter will help you save your sanity in the kitchen—and your blood sugars.

Whether it's a quick and easy Grown-Up Lunchable (page 64) or a Nutty Deconstructed Salad (page 71), all of these recipes can be ready in 15 minutes or fewer, and many don't involve any cooking at all. But the best thing about these recipes is how they can help you reduce the amount of stress in your life!

Getting dinner on the table is one of the most stressful parts of managing a home, and if you or a loved one in that home has diabetes, dinnertime can be overwhelming. And, yes, stress can raise blood sugars too.

These recipes offer simple, less stressful—but equally nourishing—options that will keep you satisfied and help promote stable blood sugars.

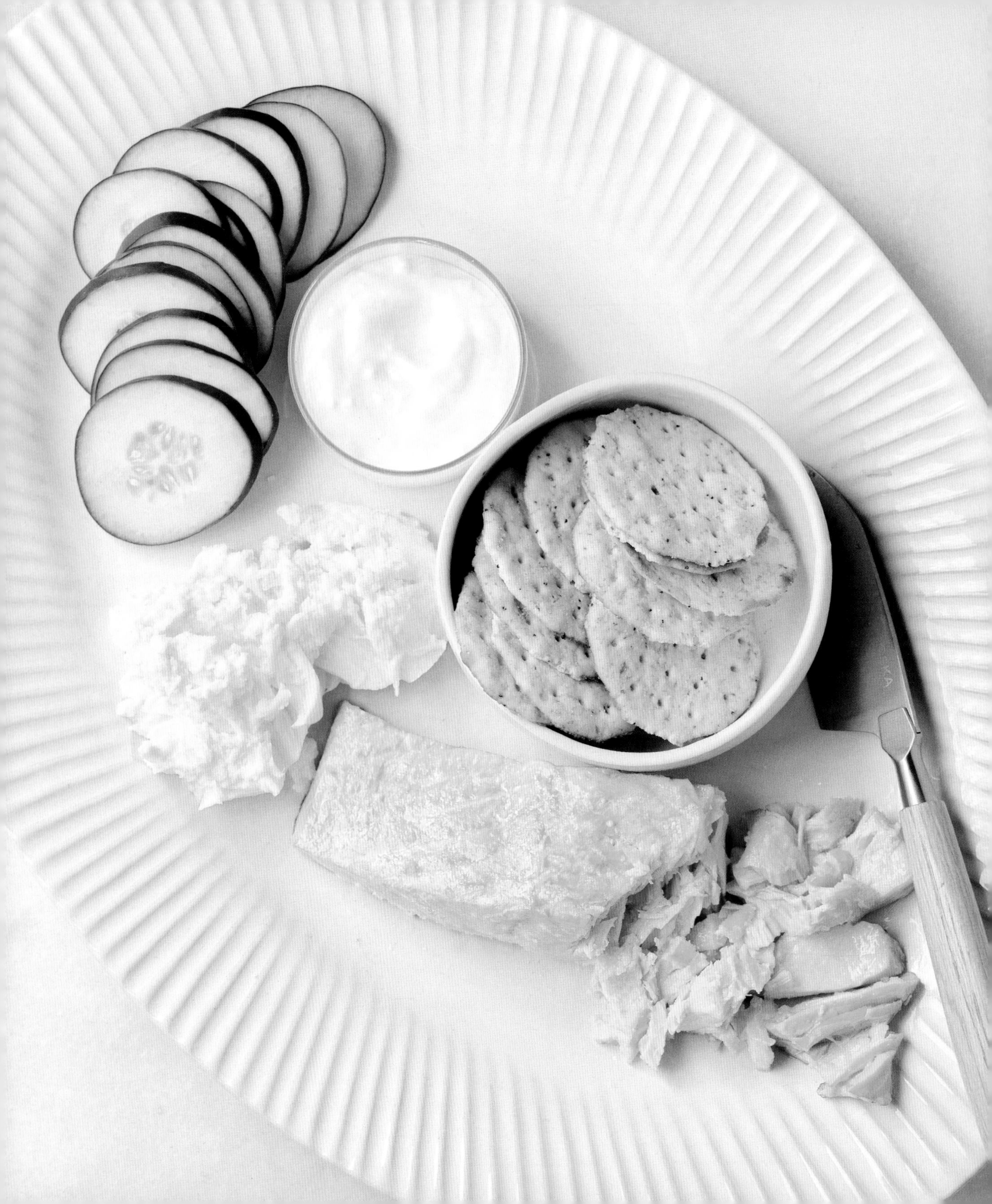

charcuterie dinner for one

This recipe turns the typical charcuterie board into a much more blood sugar–friendly option. We've swapped out processed meats for heart-healthy salmon, and we use nonfat Greek yogurt for a protein boost with less saturated fat than other dipping sauces. And—the best part—it'll be ready to eat in fewer than fifteen minutes!

no added sugar | protein packed | yield: 1 serving

1 (6-oz [170-g]) salmon fillet

Cooking oil spray, as needed

1 oz (28 g) fresh mozzarella cheese slices or balls

½ cup (60 g) thinly sliced cucumbers

¼ cup (50 g) plain nonfat Greek yogurt

1 oz (28 g) grain-free or whole-grain crackers

Preheat the oven to 400°F (204°C). Line a medium baking sheet with parchment paper.

Lightly spray the salmon fillet with the cooking oil spray and place the salmon on the prepared baking sheet. Bake the salmon for 10 to 12 minutes, or until it has browned slightly on top.

Meanwhile, assemble the mozzarella cheese, cucumbers, yogurt, and crackers on a plate.

Transfer the salmon to the plate and serve.

STORAGE: If you are making this recipe in advance, line lunch box compartments with parchment paper before adding the ingredients. Be sure to keep the foods separated. Keep the lunch box sealed tightly in the refrigerator.

Estimated Nutrition Facts per Serving: 517 calories; 16 g carbs; 1 g fiber; 5 g sugar; 47 g protein; 29 g fat (9 g saturated fat); 418 mg sodium

grown-up lunchable

Who didn't love a good cracker, meat, and cheese combo growing up? This may look like a simple snack plate, but it's actually the perfect combination of fat, fiber, and protein to help prevent blood sugar spikes after you eat—and I even included a fun low-sugar dessert too!

high fiber | protein packed | yield: 1 serving

2 oz (57 g) low-sodium, nitrate-free sliced turkey

1 oz (28 g) low-sodium sliced Swiss cheese

1 oz (28 g) grain-free or whole-grain crackers

1 tbsp (15 g) hummus

2 tbsp (30 ml) water

1 cup (30 g) arugula, baby spinach, baby kale, or other leafy green

¼ cup (30 g) sliced cucumbers or carrots

1 oz (28 g) dark chocolate

Arrange the turkey, Swiss cheese, and crackers on a plate or in a divided lunch box.

In a small bowl, combine the hummus and water, stirring them with a fork until the mixture reaches the consistency of salad dressing. (If you prefer your dressing thicker or thinner, you can adjust the water content as needed.)

In a medium bowl, toss the arugula with the hummus dressing and add it to the plate. (If you'll be eating this meal on the go, place the dressing in a small sealed container and add it to your greens just before eating.)

Top the salad with the cucumbers. Serve the dark chocolate on the side for a low-sugar treat after your meal.

STORAGE: Eat this dish immediately, or pack it in a lunch box up to 3 days in advance. Store it in a sealed container in the refrigerator.

Estimated Nutrition Facts per Serving: 512 calories; 42 g carbs; 5 g fiber; 8 g sugar; 29 g protein; 26 g fat (13 g saturated fat); 600 mg sodium

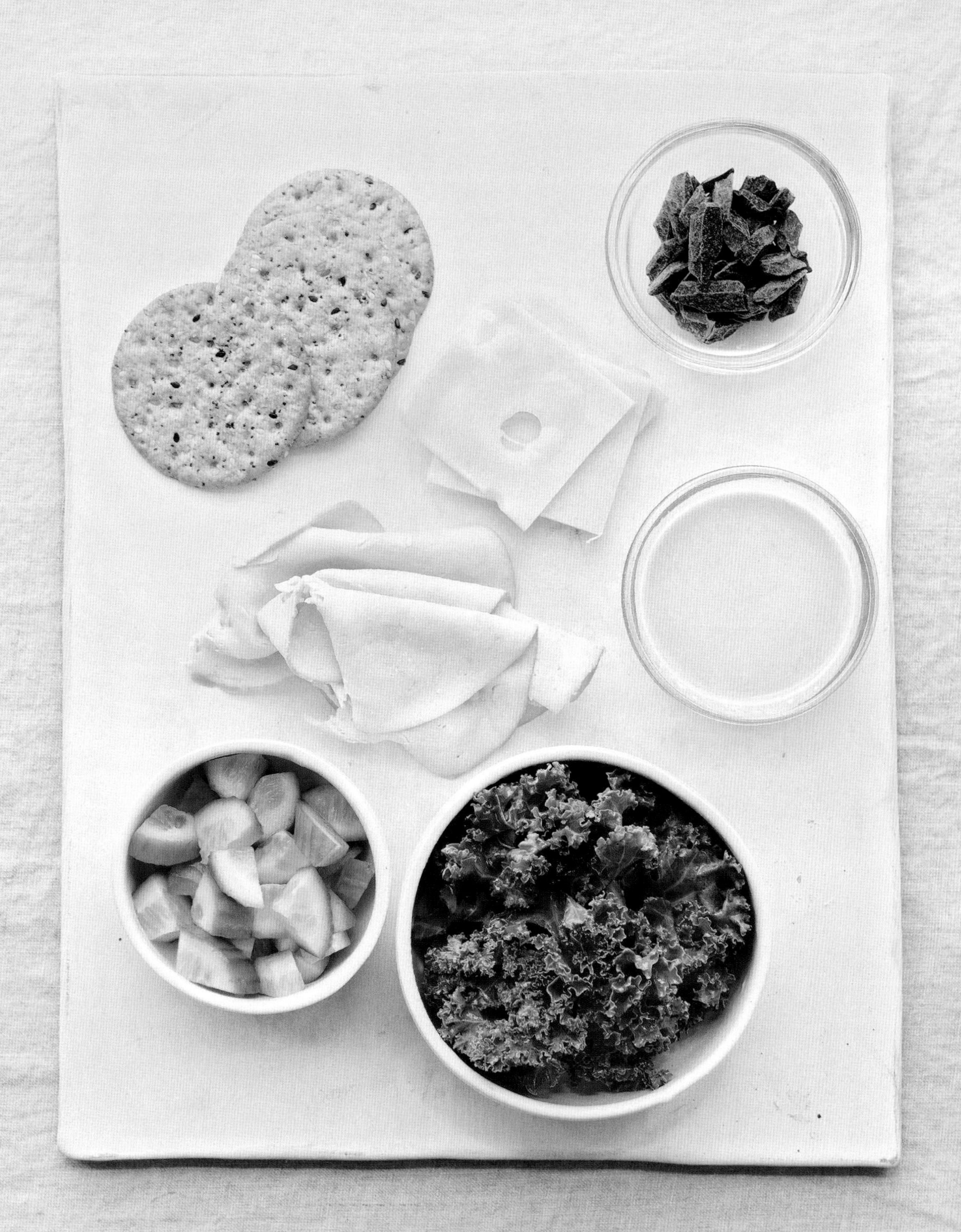

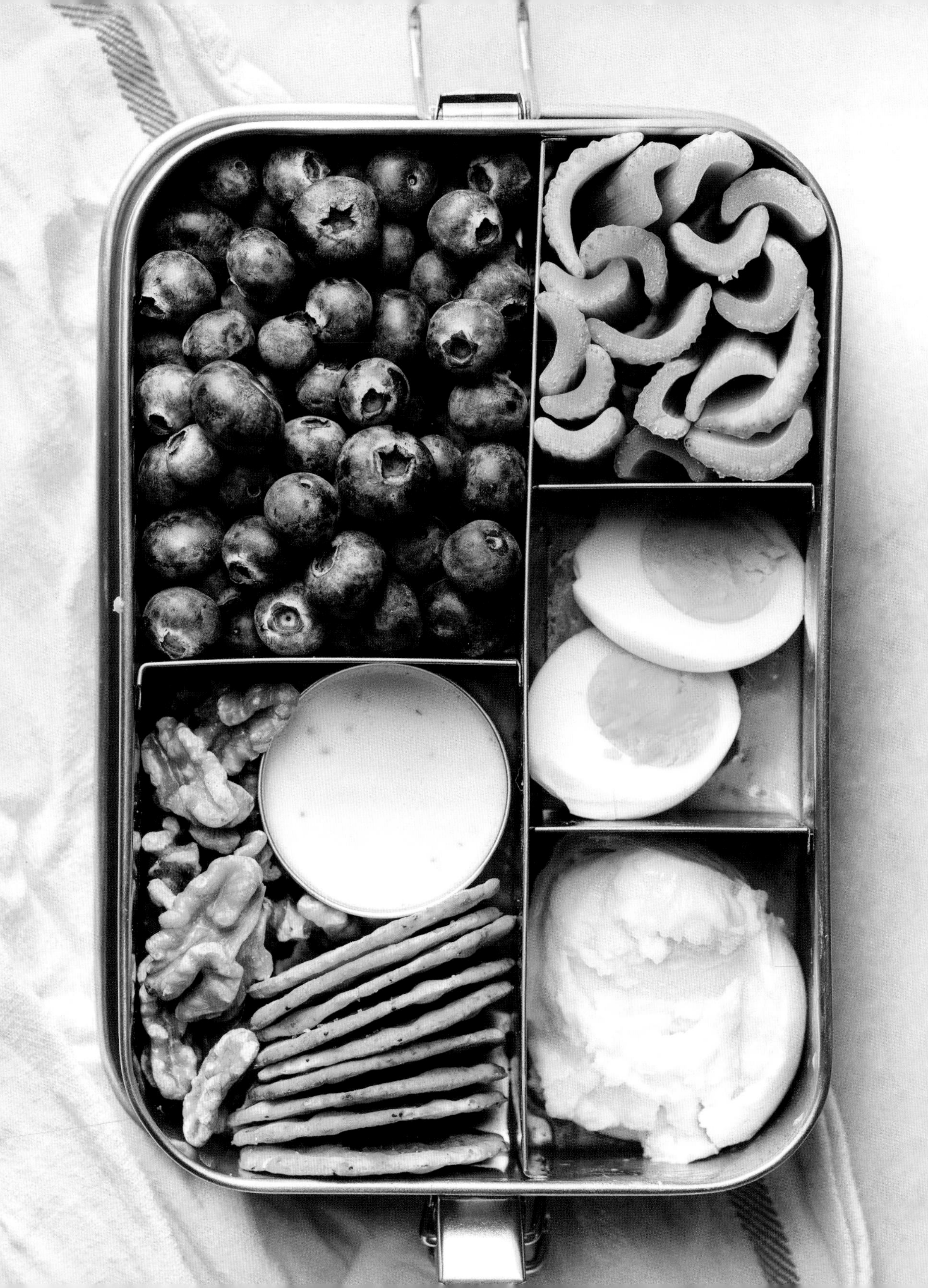

balanced bento box

This combo is the perfect meal for packing ahead of time and taking with you to work, meetings, or just for a fun meal away from the house. You don't have to use a bento box, but it certainly makes it a bit more exciting to eat! I've packed this box with the perfect amount of fat, fiber, and protein to ensure your blood sugars remain steady after you eat.

high fiber | no added sugar | protein packed | yield: 1 serving

1 oz (28 g) whole-grain or grain-free crackers

¼ cup (28 g) raw nuts of choice

1 cup (150 g) fresh blueberries

1 large hard-boiled egg

1 oz (28 g) sliced Swiss or mozzarella cheese

7 to 8 celery sticks

1 tbsp (15 ml) low-sodium salad dressing of choice

Place the crackers, nuts, blueberries, egg, Swiss cheese, celery, and salad dressing in a divided bento box if you are making the meal for later, or arrange the ingredients on a plate if you will be eating right away.

STORAGE: Pack your bento box and store it in the refrigerator for up to 3 days.

Estimated Nutrition Facts per Serving: 618 calories; 53 g carbs; 7 g fiber; 20 g sugar; 21 g protein; 38 g fat (9 g saturated fat); 516 mg sodium

fruit and veggie protein plate

You know those fancy little protein boxes you see at your favorite coffee shop? Well, this recipe will save you the $8, and it's got all the necessary fat, fiber, and protein without a ton of extra sodium, making it better for maintaining your blood sugar than the coffee shop alternative. And while grapes may typically be thought of as a no-no for people with diabetes, there's nothing to be concerned about with this recipe because we've combined them with quality fat and protein sources that will help promote stable post-meal blood sugar levels.

gluten-free | high fiber | no added sugar | protein packed | yield: 1 serving

1 cup (150 g) red seedless grapes

2 tbsp (30 g) all-natural peanut butter (see Tip)

1 large hard-boiled egg

1 oz (28 g) cubed Cheddar cheese

10 to 15 baby carrots

Place the grapes, peanut butter, egg, Cheddar cheese, and carrots in a lunch box if you are making the meal for later, or arrange the ingredients on a plate if you will be eating right away.

STORAGE: You can pack and store this meal up to 3 days in advance. Just make sure to store it in a sealed container in the refrigerator.

TIP: Be sure to buy an all-natural peanut butter with no added salt or sugar.

Estimated Nutrition Facts per Serving: 526 calories; 45 g carbs; 5 g fiber; 33 g sugar; 23 g protein; 31 g fat (11 g saturated fat); 340 mg sodium

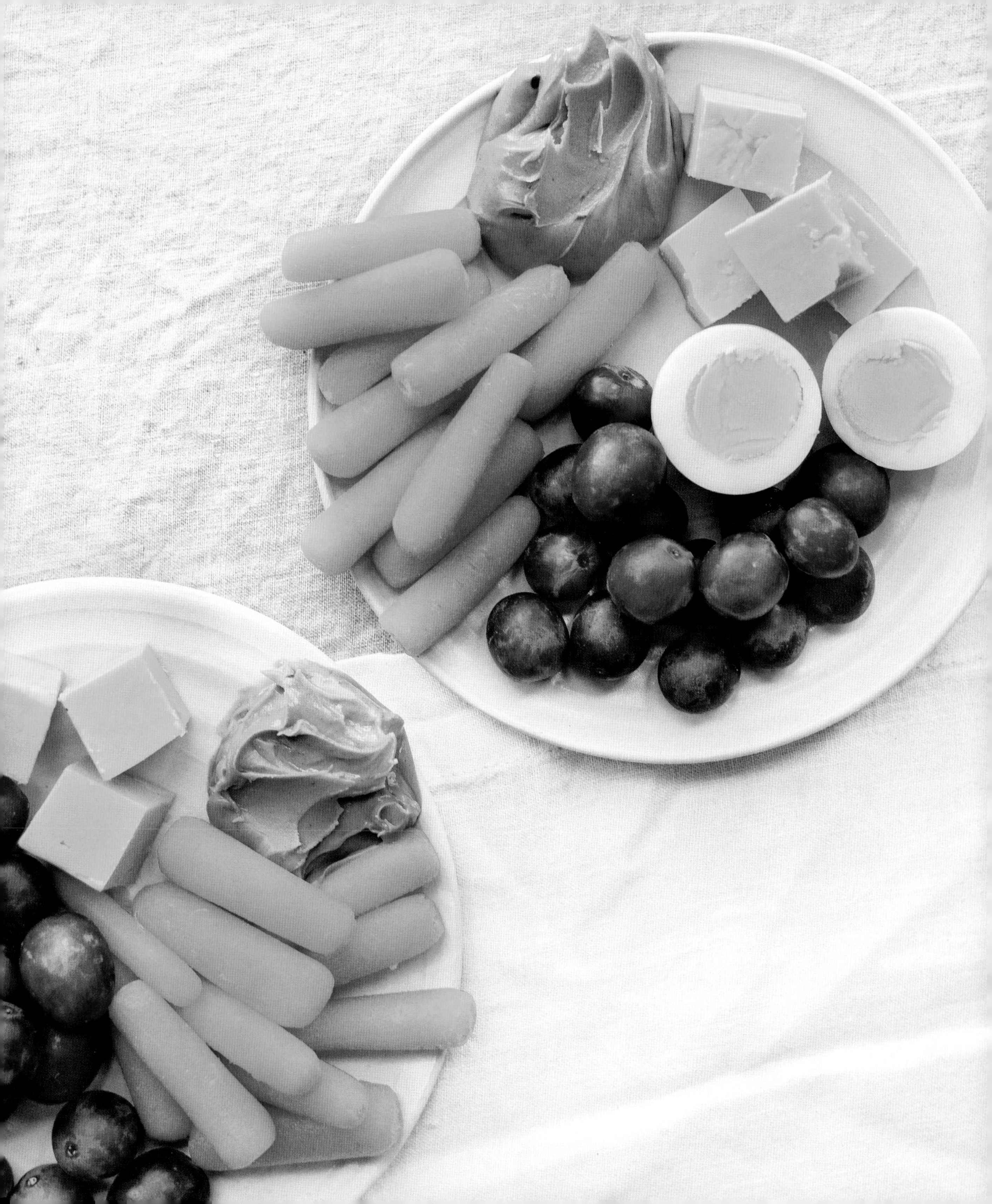

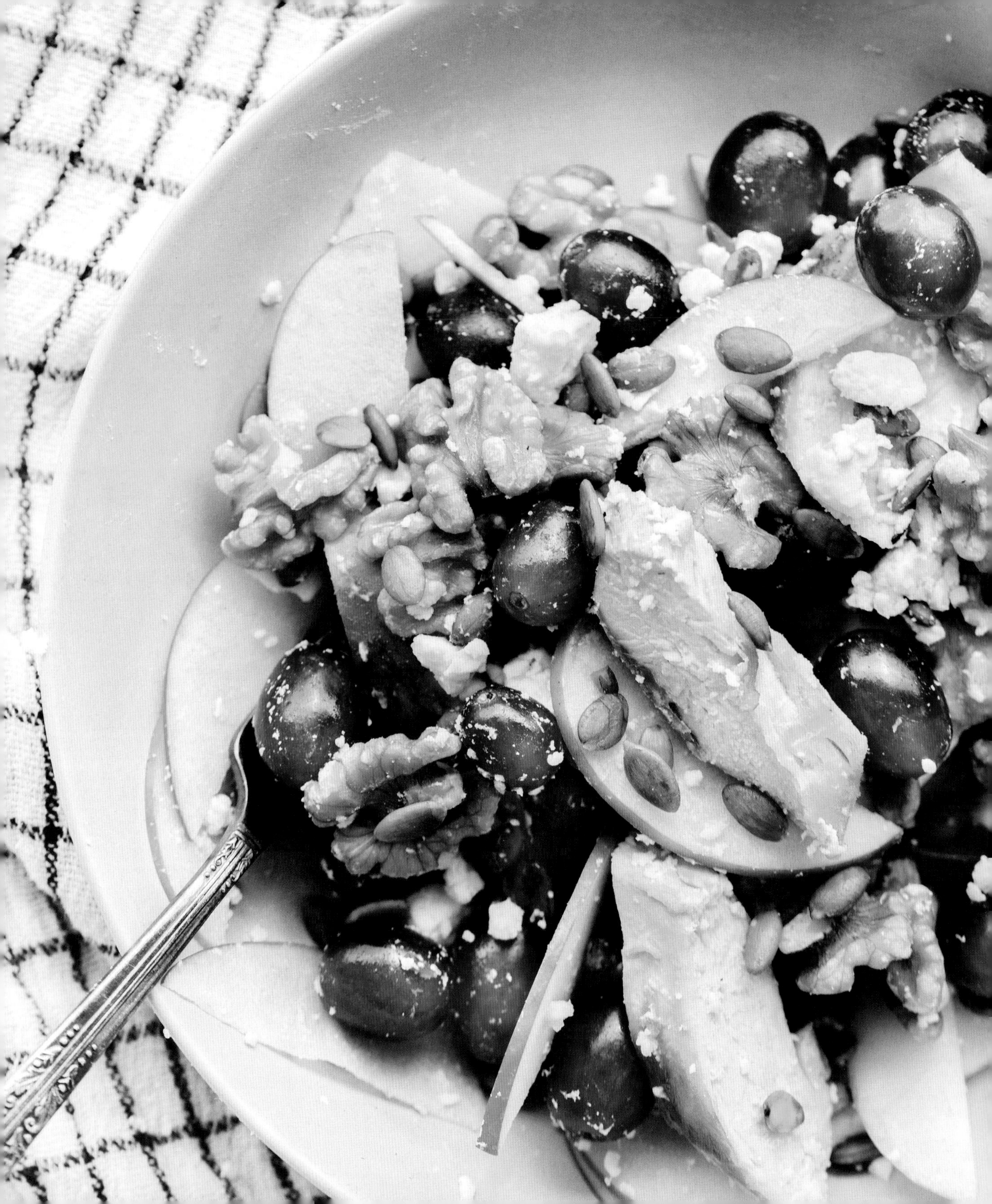

nutty deconstructed salad

Imagine your favorite salad with all the best flavors—but without the lettuce, which will wilt if stored as leftovers—and you've got this Nutty Deconstructed Salad! It's loaded with quality fat and protein sources to keep you full and satisfied and your blood sugars happy. Many salad dressings are often loaded with hidden sugars, but with this perfect combination of salad toppings, there's no need for extra dressing!

gluten-free | high fiber | no added sugar | protein packed | yield: 1 serving

6 oz (170 g) grilled or baked chicken, sliced or cubed to the desired size

½ cup (75 g) red seedless grapes

¼ cup (32 g) crumbled feta cheese

¼ cup (30 g) raw walnuts

2 tbsp (10 g) raw pumpkin seeds

1 small apple, thinly sliced

In a salad bowl, combine the chicken, grapes, feta cheese, walnuts, pumpkin seeds, and apple. Toss to combine the ingredients and serve.

STORAGE: Store the deconstructed salad in a sealed container in the refrigerator for up to 3 days.

> TIP: To keep this meal under the 15-minute prep time, I always keep precooked chicken breasts in my freezer. You can find some great low-sodium, precooked options in the freezer section of your local grocery store.

Estimated Nutrition Facts per Serving: 613 calories; 42 g carbs; 6 g fiber; 30 g sugar; 42 g protein; 33 g fat (10 g saturated fat); 501 mg sodium

mediterranean pasta salad with goat cheese

This pasta salad is a diabetes-friendly option to traditional pasta salad. It's loaded with veggies, fiber, and flavor, and it packs a great protein punch since it calls for bean-based pasta. It's also great for meal prep on the weekends, so you can eat it throughout the week!

gluten-free | high fiber | no added sugar | protein packed | yield: 4 servings

½ cup (75 g) grape tomatoes, sliced in half lengthwise

1 medium red bell pepper, coarsely chopped

½ medium red onion, sliced into thin strips

1 medium zucchini, coarsely chopped

1 cup (175 g) broccoli florets

½ cup (110 g) oil-packed artichoke hearts, drained

¼ cup (60 ml) olive oil

½ tsp sea salt

½ tsp black pepper

1 tbsp (3 g) dried oregano

½ tsp garlic powder

4 oz (113 g) crumbled goat cheese

½ cup (50 g) shaved Parmesan cheese

8 oz (227 g) lentil or chickpea penne pasta, cooked, rinsed, and drained

In a large bowl, combine the tomatoes, bell pepper, onion, zucchini, broccoli, artichoke hearts, oil, sea salt, black pepper, oregano, garlic powder, goat cheese, and Parmesan cheese. Gently mix everything together to combine and coat all of the ingredients with the oil.

Add the pasta to the bowl and stir to combine.

Let the pasta salad rest for 1 to 2 hours in the refrigerator to marinate it, or serve the pasta salad immediately if desired.

Storage: Store the pasta salad in a sealed container in the refrigerator for up to 5 days.

TIPS: To save even more time when preparing the recipe, make sure to chop your veggies ahead of time or purchase precut veggies. They can save a ton of time in the kitchen!

Squeeze some fresh lemon juice on top of the salad just before serving for an added burst of freshness!

Estimated Nutrition Facts per Serving: 477 calories; 41 g carbs; 6 g fiber; 6 g sugar; 23 g protein; 24 g fat (8 g saturated fat); 706 mg sodium

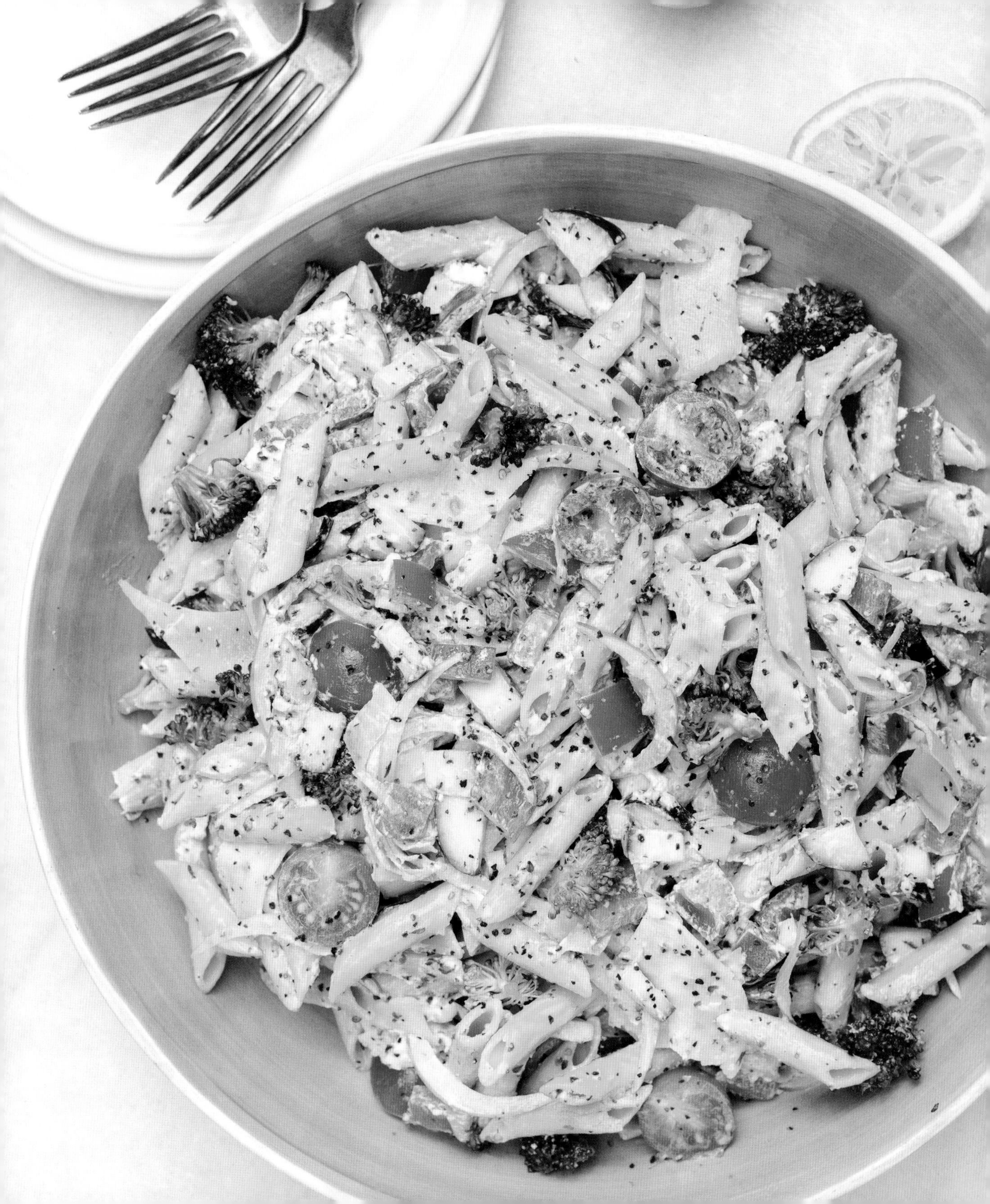

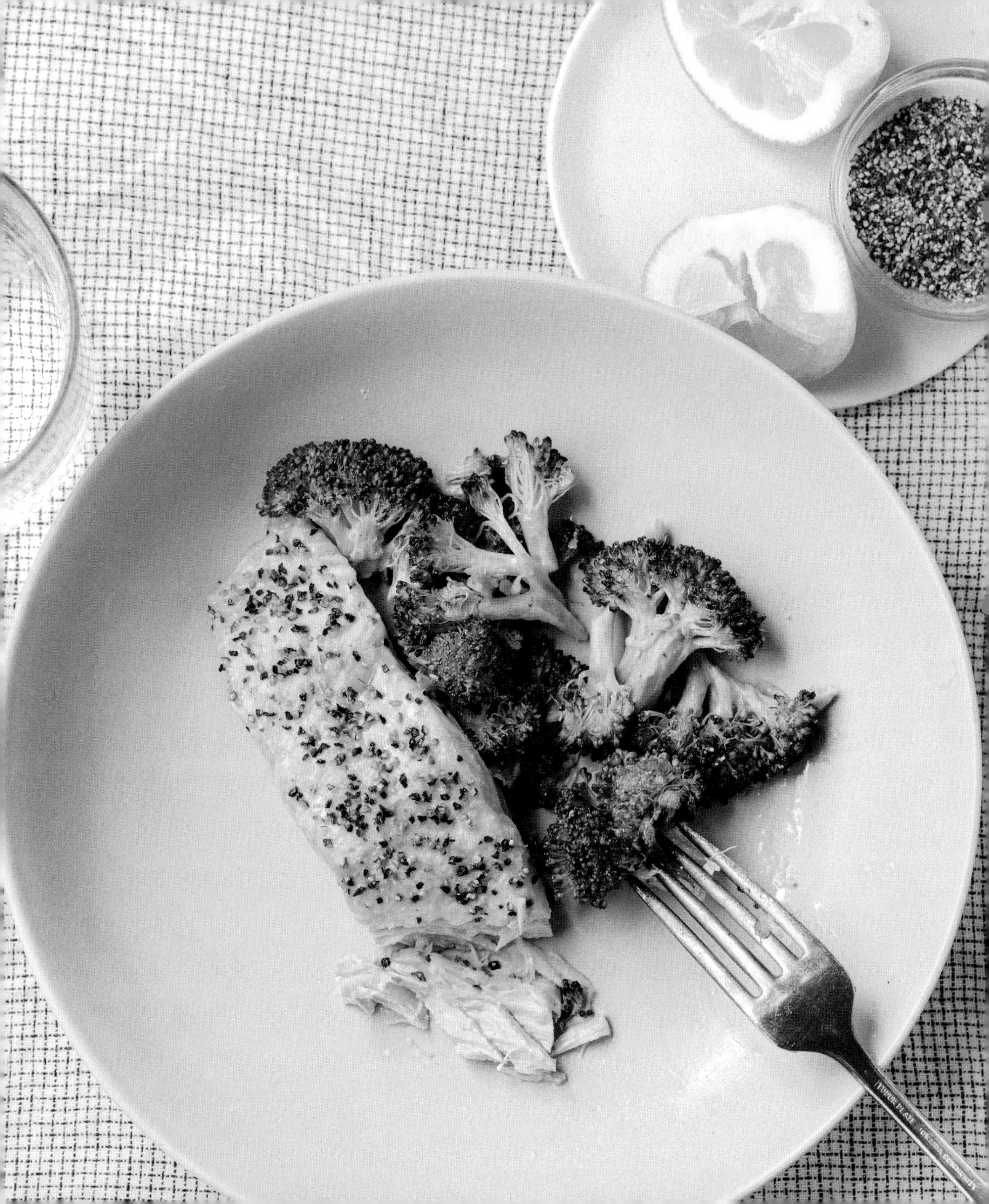

lemon-pepper salmon with roasted broccoli

Many people are intimidated by the thought of cooking fish, but it's actually one of the quickest and easiest meal options out there. I love salmon because it's loaded with better-for-you fats and protein. People with diabetes are at a greater risk of developing heart disease, so it's important to make food choices that protect your heart. The American Heart Association recommends eating seafood two times per week to help support a healthy heart!

gluten-free | low carb | no added sugar | protein packed | yield: 4 servings

4 (6-oz [170-g]) salmon fillets

Cooking oil spray, as needed

Juice of 1 medium lemon (see Tips)

½ tsp black pepper

¼ tsp garlic salt or ¼ tsp sea salt mixed with ¼ tsp garlic powder

1 lb (454 g) broccoli florets

¼ tsp sea salt

¼ tsp garlic powder

Preheat the oven to 400°F (204°C). Line two large baking sheets with parchment paper.

Place the salmon on the first prepared baking sheet, making sure the fillets are evenly spaced. Spray the salmon with the cooking oil spray. Drizzle the lemon juice over each of the salmon fillets, then sprinkle the black pepper and garlic salt over each fillet.

Spread the broccoli out evenly on the second prepared baking sheet and spray the broccoli with cooking oil spray. Sprinkle the sea salt and garlic powder over the broccoli.

Place both baking sheets in the oven. Bake the salmon for 10 to 12 minutes, until it is light brown, depending on your preferred doneness and the thickness of the fillets. Bake the broccoli for 12 minutes, until the edges are slightly crispy. Serve the salmon and broccoli immediately.

STORAGE: The salmon can be kept in a sealed container in the refrigerator for up to 2 days. The broccoli can be kept in a sealed container in the refrigerator for up to 7 days.

TIPS: I like my salmon very lemony, but if you prefer a little less zing, you can use the juice of just half of the lemon.

If this is not enough food to fill you up and keep you satisfied, you can definitely add a piece of whole-grain toast or a few whole-grain crackers for some quick and easy whole-grain carbohydrate goodness.

Estimated Nutrition Facts per Serving: 353 calories; 9 g carbs; 3 g fiber; 2 g sugar; 37 g protein; 19 g fat (4 g saturated fat); 406 mg sodium

pesto pasta in a pinch

This dish is a higher-protein, lower-carbohydrate pasta dish that will have you loving pasta again! It is perfect for busy weeknights or meal prepping on the weekend. It's quite simple, but it's still loaded with plant-based fats and protein. You can add poultry, meat, or tofu if you'd like an extra protein boost, but because we use a bean-based pasta, it's already loaded with protein to keep you fuller longer and keep your blood sugars balanced.

gluten-free | high fiber | no added sugar | sodium aware | yield: 4 servings

½ cup (12 g) fresh basil leaves

½ cup (15 g) baby spinach

2 tbsp (14 g) coarsely chopped walnuts

½ tbsp (5 g) minced garlic

¼ cup (60 ml) olive oil

¼ cup (32 g) crumbled feta cheese

8 oz (227 g) chickpea or lentil pasta, cooked

1 cup (149 g) halved grape tomatoes

In a food processor or blender, combine the basil, spinach, walnuts, garlic, oil, and feta cheese. Process the ingredients for 30 to 45 seconds, until they are homogeneous.

Place the pasta in a medium bowl. Pour the pesto over the pasta and toss to coat it in the sauce.

Gently fold in the tomatoes, then serve the pasta.

STORAGE: Store the pasta in a sealed container in the refrigerator for up to 5 days.

TIPS: You can also use a store-bought pesto sauce, but be sure to look for a variety with a low amount of sodium and quality ingredients.

Add freshly ground black pepper to the pesto sauce to add some kick to it!

Estimated Nutrition Facts per Serving: 374 calories; 38 g carbs; 6 g fiber; 2 g sugar; 13 g protein; 21 g fat (4 g saturated fat); 139 mg sodium

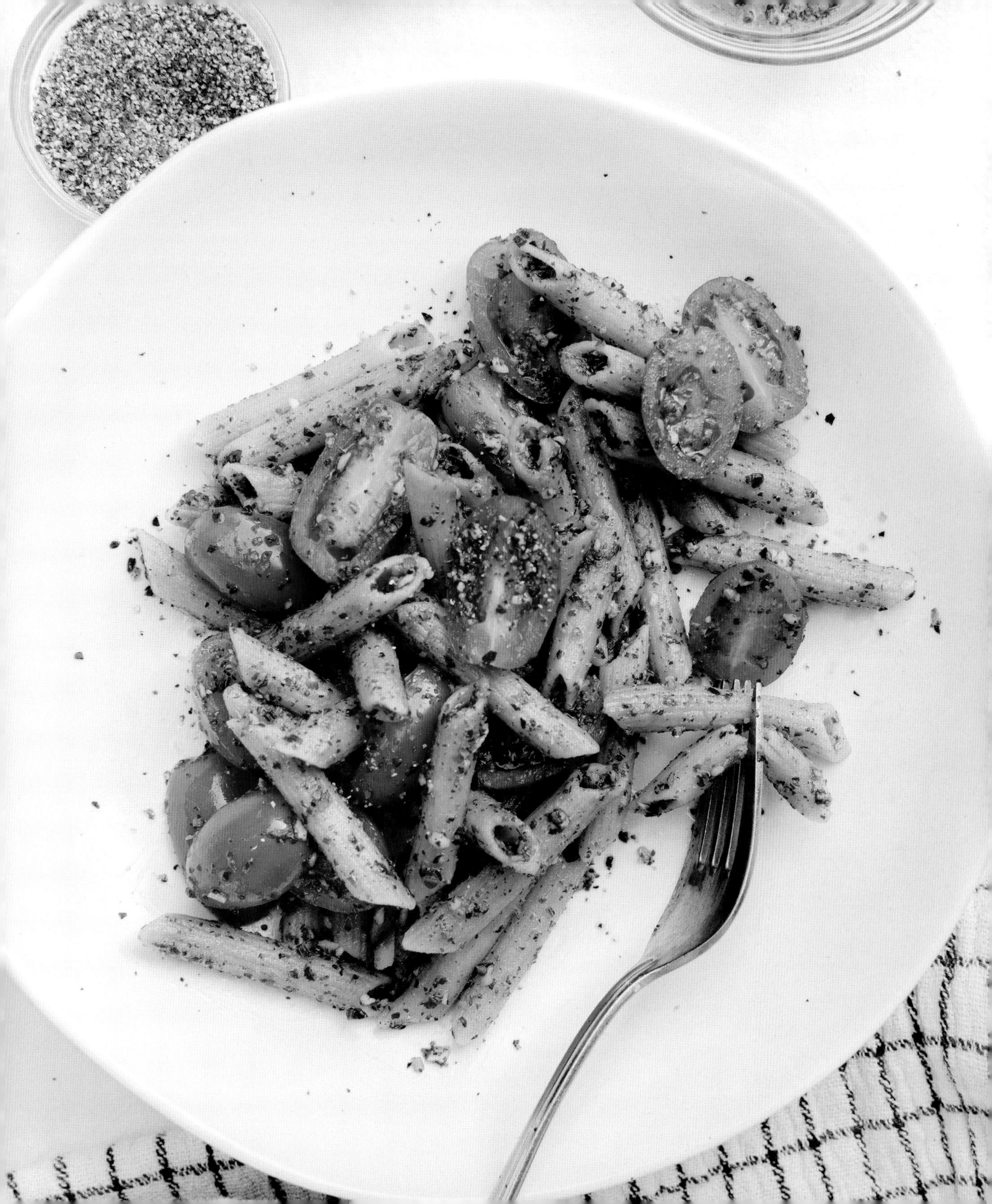

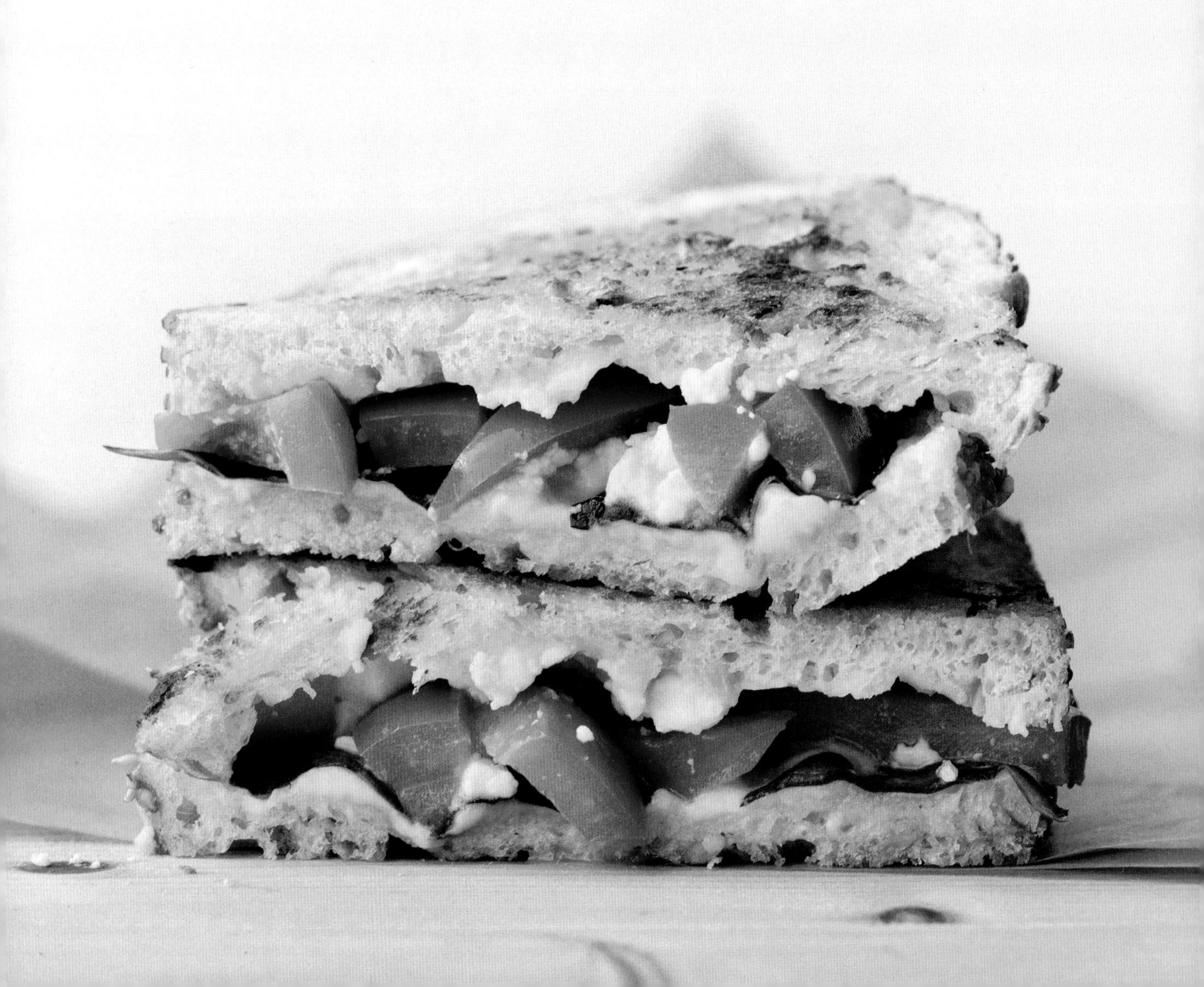

veggie grilled cheese sandwich

I'll take any opportunity to add veggies to a dish. Adding veggies not only increases our vitamin and mineral intake but it also increases the amount of fiber in a dish. And remember: Fiber helps balance blood sugars! This Veggie Grilled Cheese Sandwich is loaded with flavor and deliciousness and offers a great way to sneak more veggies in! Serve it with your favorite fruit or some more veggies and you've got an easy, delicious dinner.

high fiber | no added sugar | protein packed | yield: 1 serving

Cooking oil spray, as needed

2 slices whole-grain bread

1 oz (28 g) shredded mozzarella cheese

¼ cup (8 g) baby spinach

5 to 6 thin strips red bell pepper

2 tbsp (16 g) crumbled feta cheese

Spray a medium skillet with cooking oil spray. Heat the skillet over medium heat.

Lightly spray each side of both slices of bread with the cooking oil spray.

Place 1 slice of bread in the skillet and carefully layer on the ingredients in this order: mozzarella cheese, spinach, bell pepper, feta cheese, second slice of bread.

Cook the sandwich for about 4 minutes, until the cheeses begin to melt.

Carefully flip the sandwich and cook it for 3 to 4 minutes on the opposite side. Serve the sandwich immediately.

STORAGE: Eat this sandwich immediately, as it does not keep well.

TIP: Add some caramelized onions for even more flavor!

Estimated Nutrition Facts per Serving: 339 calories; 39 g carbs; 5 g fiber; 8 g sugar; 21 g protein; 13 g fat (7 g saturated fat); 729 mg sodium

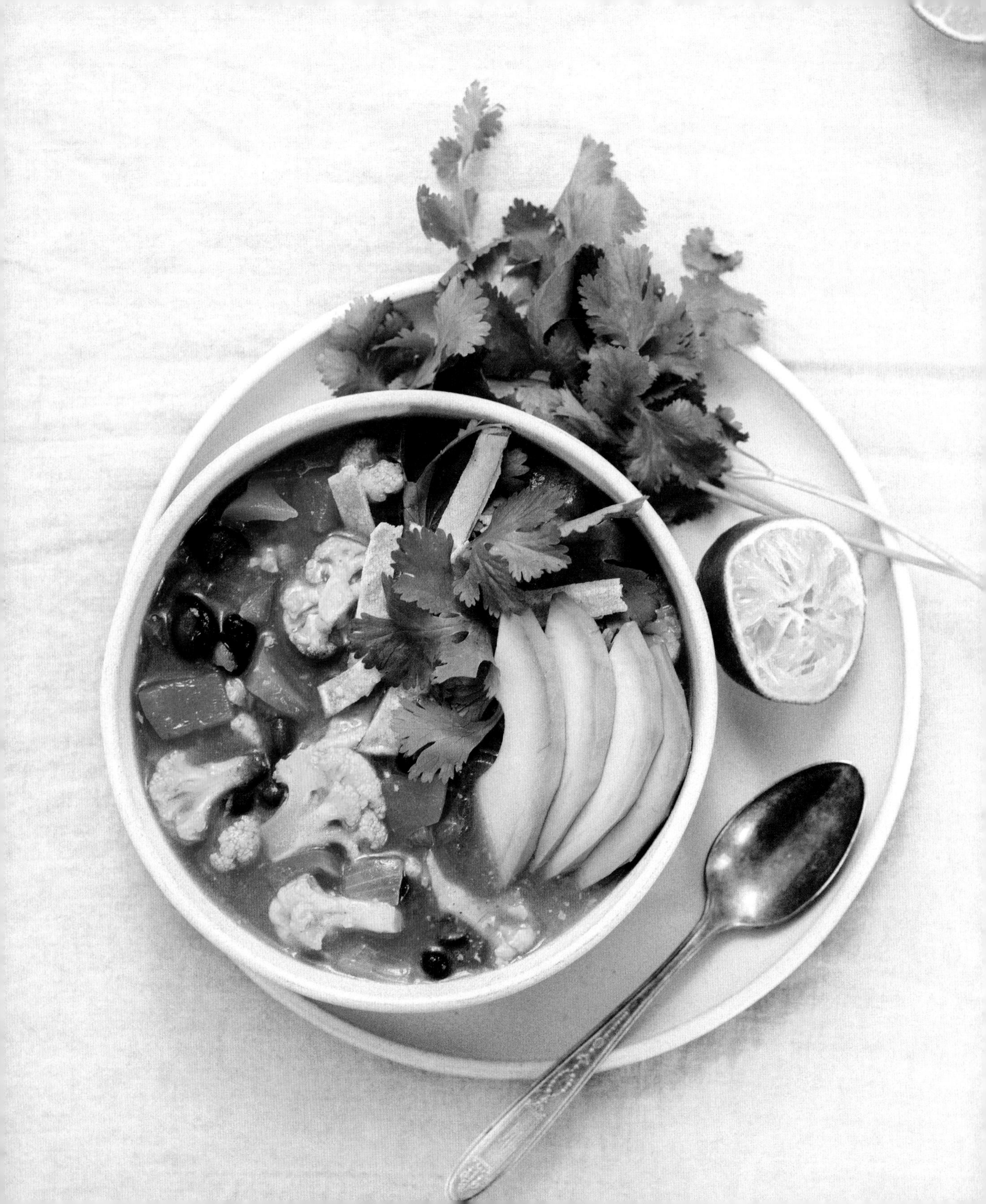

nourishing soups and salads

ONE-POT AND ONE-BOWL MEALS EVERYONE CAN ENJOY

Soups and salads are perfect for easy weeknight meals, and these recipes are ideal for helping you balance your blood sugars throughout the day with simple and easy one-pot or one-bowl options. Each of these recipes is a careful balance of fat, fiber, and protein and will help relieve some of that dinnertime stress that creeps up when life gets hectic.

Soups can be made ahead of time on the weekend and eaten throughout the week for lunch or dinner. And believe it or not, you can prepare salads ahead of time too. Simply prep all of your toppings and dressings on the weekend, or whenever works for your schedule. Wait until right before you're ready to eat to toss your greens in any dressing—otherwise, the rest of the ingredients can be prepped ahead of time.

A note on soups, salads, and blood sugars: Many soup and salad recipes can actually be hard on blood sugars, but for different reasons. Soups often contain traditionally higher-carbohydrate ingredients like pasta, rice, and potatoes. These can potentially spike blood sugars more than you'd like. And salads often have very few carbohydrates in them, which can actually lead to low blood sugars a few hours later. Eating some amount of carbohydrates at each meal and snack is essential for maintaining stable blood sugar levels, and often medications are dosed assuming you're eating some carbohydrates at each meal. While it's important to not eat too many carbohydrates when you have diabetes, it's also important to make sure you're getting enough. It's about balance.

So, instead of taking pasta, rice, and potatoes out of soups—because let's be honest, they are delicious—I've paired them with some scrumptious veggies and other ingredients that help lower carbs' impact on your blood sugars. And I've added some naturally blood sugar–friendly carbohydrate sources to your favorite salad recipes to help keep things nice and steady.

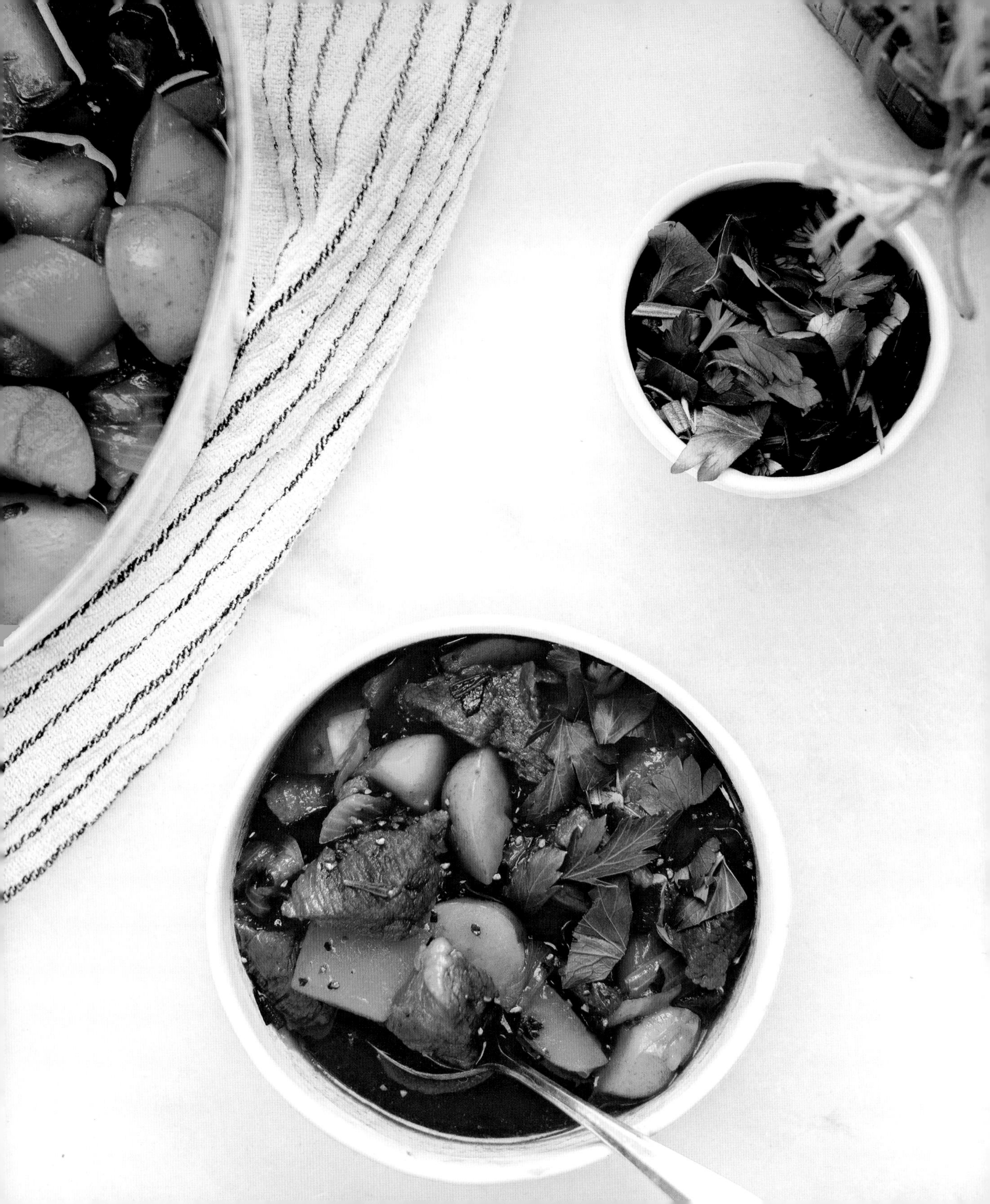

hearty beef and veggie stew

This beef stew is perfect for chilly afternoons or evenings. It's loaded with flavor and fiber-filled, satisfying veggies! The added fiber in this stew makes it a blood sugar–friendly alternative to traditional beef stew. And did I mention it can be ready to eat in under an hour?

gluten-free | high fiber | no added sugar | protein packed | yield: 4 servings

2 tbsp (30 ml) avocado oil

1 lb (454 g) extra lean beef stew meat

1 medium yellow onion, cut into large chunks

4 large carrots, cut into 2-inch (5-cm) chunks

5 to 6 small red potatoes, quartered

3 cups (720 ml) low-sodium beef broth

½ tsp salt

½ tsp black pepper

¼ to ⅓ cup (16 to 21 g) finely chopped fresh herbs of choice (see Tip)

Heat the oil in a large Dutch oven or pot over medium-high heat.

Add the stew meat and cook it for 2 to 3 minutes on each side, until it is brown on all sides but still pink in the center. Remove the stew meat from the Dutch oven and set it aside.

Add the onion and carrots to the Dutch oven and cook them for 5 to 10 minutes, until they start to soften.

Add the potatoes, broth, salt, black pepper, and herbs. Bring the mixture to a boil. Reduce the heat to low and simmer the stew for 30 minutes, until the vegetables are fork-tender.

Add the stew meat to the stew and cook it for 5 to 10 minutes to warm the meat through. Serve the stew immediately.

STORAGE: Enjoy this stew immediately, or let it cool in the refrigerator and then freeze it in individual portions for up to 3 months.

TIP: For this recipe, I like to use parsley, rosemary, and basil.

Estimated Nutrition Facts per Serving: 400 calories; 45 g carbs; 6 g fiber; 8 g sugar; 32 g protein; 11 g fat (2 g saturated fat); 742 mg sodium

high-fiber pumpkin-cashew soup

A creamy soup that gets its richness from fiber-rich beans and cashews? Count me in! This soup comes together in fewer than 15 minutes and supplies about one-third of your daily fiber intake per serving. Remember, fiber not only helps keep you fuller longer but it also promotes more balanced blood sugar numbers after you eat.

gluten-free | high fiber | no added sugar | sodium aware | vegan | yield: 4 servings

1 tbsp (15 ml) olive oil

3 medium carrots, coarsely chopped

1 medium onion, coarsely chopped

1 tbsp (6 g) grated fresh ginger or ¼ tsp ground ginger

1 tsp ground cinnamon

½ tsp ground cumin

½ tsp ground nutmeg

1 (15-oz [425-g]) can pumpkin purée

2 cups (480 ml) low-sodium vegetable broth

1 cup (240 ml) plain unsweetened almond milk

½ cup (55 g) raw cashews

½ (15-oz [425-g]) can navy beans, undrained

1 tsp apple cider vinegar

Heat the oil in a large pot over medium heat.

Add the carrots, onion, ginger, cinnamon, cumin, and nutmeg. Sauté this mixture for 5 to 7 minutes, or until the onion is translucent.

Add the pumpkin purée, broth, and almond milk and stir to combine.

Simmer the soup for 15 minutes, or until the carrots are soft.

Let the soup cool slightly, then transfer it to a high-power blender and add the cashews, beans and their liquid, and vinegar. Blend the soup until it is smooth and creamy.

Serve the soup immediately, or freeze it in smaller portions for future use.

STORAGE: Freeze this soup for up to 3 months, or store it in a sealed container in the refrigerator for up to 7 days.

Estimated Nutrition Facts per Serving: 260 calories; 34 g carbs; 9 g fiber; 11 g sugar; 9 g protein; 12 g fat (2 g saturated fat); 152 mg sodium

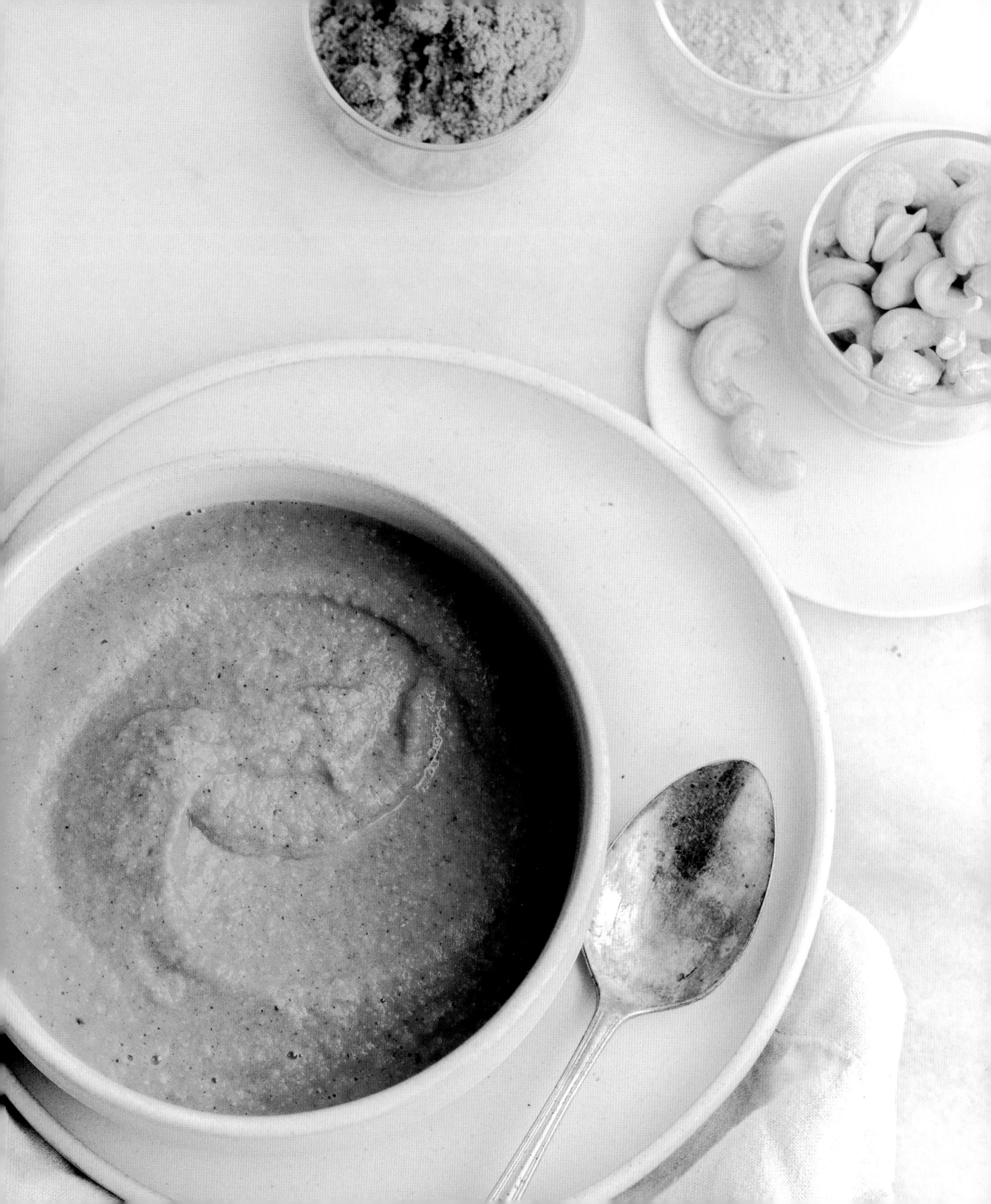

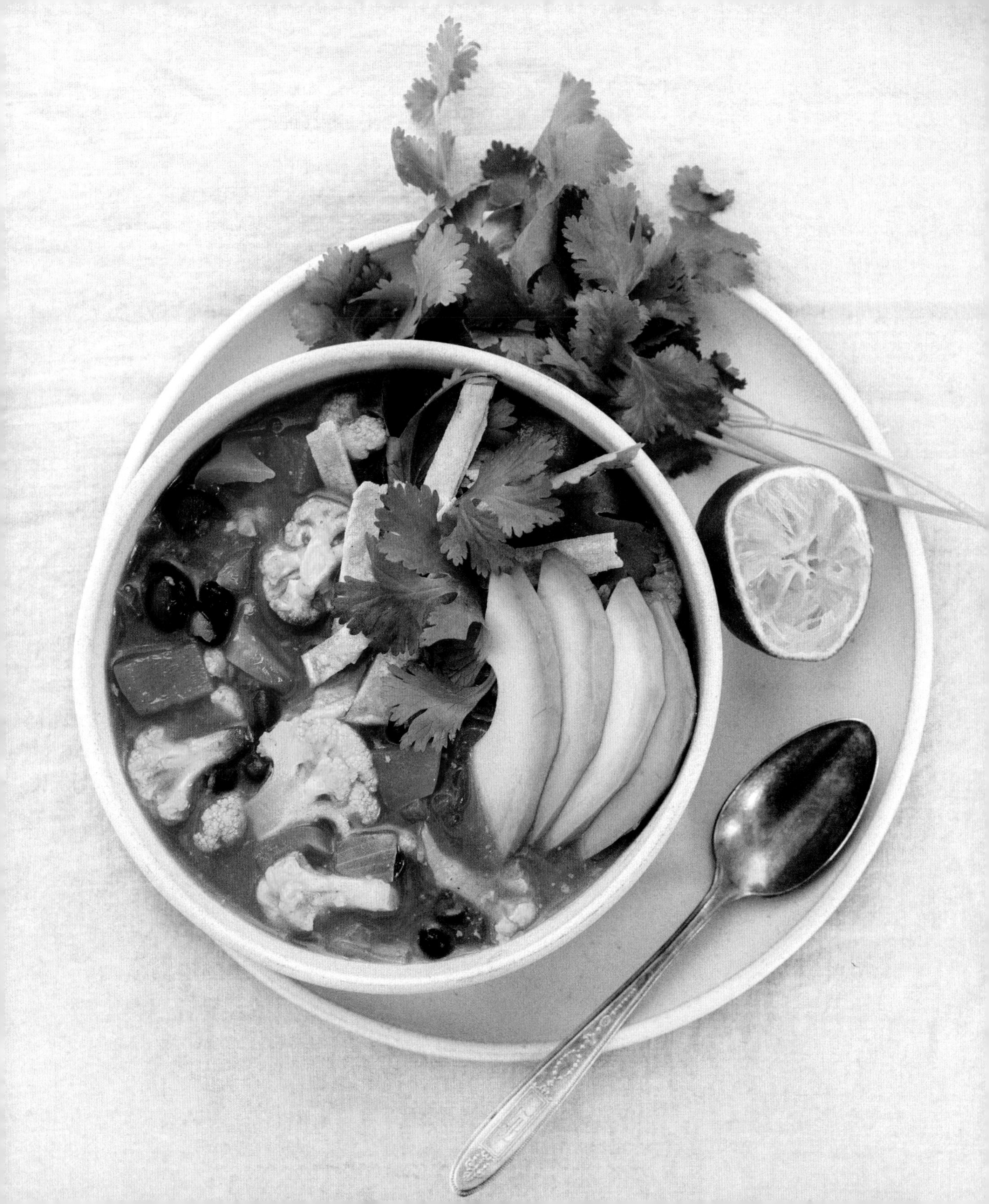

black bean, turmeric, and cauliflower tortilla soup

Think of this recipe as your favorite quesadilla transformed into a comforting, high-fiber veggie soup! While you could streamline the recipe by adding the raw cauliflower to the pot and simmering it with the spices, I think it's well worth the extra step of roasting it to achieve that delicious flavor. The carbohydrate count in this soup may seem like too much for someone with diabetes, but the fiber and protein help slow down how quickly your body absorbs those carbohydrates, making it much more blood sugar–friendly than traditional tortilla soup!

gluten-free | high fiber | no added sugar | yield: 4 servings

1 medium head cauliflower, chopped into medium florets

2 tsp (10 ml) extra virgin olive oil, divided

½ tsp ground turmeric

½ tsp garlic powder

1 medium yellow onion, coarsely chopped

1 clove garlic, minced

1 medium red bell pepper, coarsely chopped

2 cups (480 ml) low-sodium salsa

1 tsp chipotle chili powder (see Tips)

4 cups (960 ml) water

Juice of ½ medium lime

1 (15-oz [425-g]) can black beans, drained and rinsed

½ cup (60 g) shredded Cheddar cheese

Finely chopped fresh cilantro, as needed

Avocado, sliced (optional)

4 lime wedges

Preheat the oven to 425°F (218°C).

Place the cauliflower florets in a large bowl. Add 1 teaspoon of the oil, turmeric, and garlic powder and toss the cauliflower florets to coat them in the seasonings. Transfer the cauliflower to a large baking sheet. Bake the cauliflower for 25 minutes, until it is golden brown.

Meanwhile, heat the remaining 1 teaspoon of oil in a large pot over medium heat. Add the onion, garlic, and bell pepper and sauté the vegetables for 5 to 10 minutes, or until the onion is translucent with charred edges. Add the salsa, chipotle chili powder, water, lime juice, and black beans and bring the soup to a simmer.

When the cauliflower is done, add it and the Cheddar cheese to the soup. Simmer the soup for at least 15 to 20 minutes to allow the flavors to meld.

Serve the soup with the cilantro sprinkled on top, avocado if desired, and a lime wedge on the side of each serving.

STORAGE: Freeze the soup for up to 3 months, or store it in a sealed container in the refrigerator for up to 7 days.

TIPS: Look for salsas that have less than 100 milligrams of sodium per serving. If you prefer a milder soup, reduce or omit the chipotle chili powder.

Estimated Nutrition Facts per Serving: 347 calories; 62 g carbs; 13 g fiber; 15 g sugar; 13 g protein; 7 g fat (2 g saturated fat); 268 mg sodium

coconut, miso, and sweet potato white bean chili

This crowd-pleasing chili gets a makeover from the East with a coconut-miso broth and sesame-scallion tempeh crumbles. Not only is it impressive to your taste buds but it also boasts nearly half of your daily recommended fiber intake and 22 grams of plant-based protein per serving!

high fiber | no added sugar | protein packed | vegan | yield: 4 servings

2 tsp (10 ml) sesame oil, divided

1 medium white onion, coarsely chopped

2 tsp (6 g) minced fresh garlic

2 tsp (4 g) grated fresh ginger

1 tbsp (17 g) miso of choice dissolved in 3 tbsp (45 ml) warm water (see Tips)

1 (14-oz [397-ml]) can light coconut milk

2 cups (480 ml) water

2 medium sweet potatoes, cubed

1 (15-oz [425-g]) can navy beans, drained and rinsed

8 oz (227 g) tempeh, crumbled (see Tips)

2 green onions, finely chopped

2 tbsp (30 ml) low-sodium tamari

3 cups (200 g) coarsely chopped kale

1 pinch of cayenne pepper (optional)

Sea salt, as needed

Black pepper, as needed

Heat 1 teaspoon of the oil in a large pot over medium heat. Add the onion, garlic, and ginger and sauté the mixture for about 5 minutes, or until the edges of the onion start to caramelize.

Add the miso-water mixture, coconut milk, water, sweet potatoes, and beans to the pot. Cover the pot and simmer the chili for about 30 minutes, or until the sweet potatoes are fork-tender.

Meanwhile, heat the remaining 1 teaspoon of oil in a medium skillet over medium heat. Add the tempeh, green onions, and tamari. Cook the mixture for 7 to 10 minutes, or until the tempeh is crispy.

Stir the tempeh mixture, kale, cayenne pepper (if using), sea salt, and black pepper into the chili, then serve.

STORAGE: Freeze the chili for up to 3 months, or store it in a sealed container in the refrigerator for up to 7 days.

TIPS: Miso is a fermented soybean paste popular in Asian cuisines and used to give umami flavor to dishes. You can find it near the tofu in your local grocery store, in health food stores, or online. Miso comes in white, yellow, and red varieties. The darker the color, the more pungent the taste.

Tempeh is a soy-based protein found in the same refrigerated section of the grocery store as tofu. However, unlike tofu, tempeh is most often made from fermented soybeans, which forms a condensed, solid structure.

Estimated Nutrition Facts per Serving: 407 calories; 45 g carbs; 12 g fiber; 5 g sugar; 22 g protein; 16 g fat (8 g saturated fat); 1,134 mg sodium

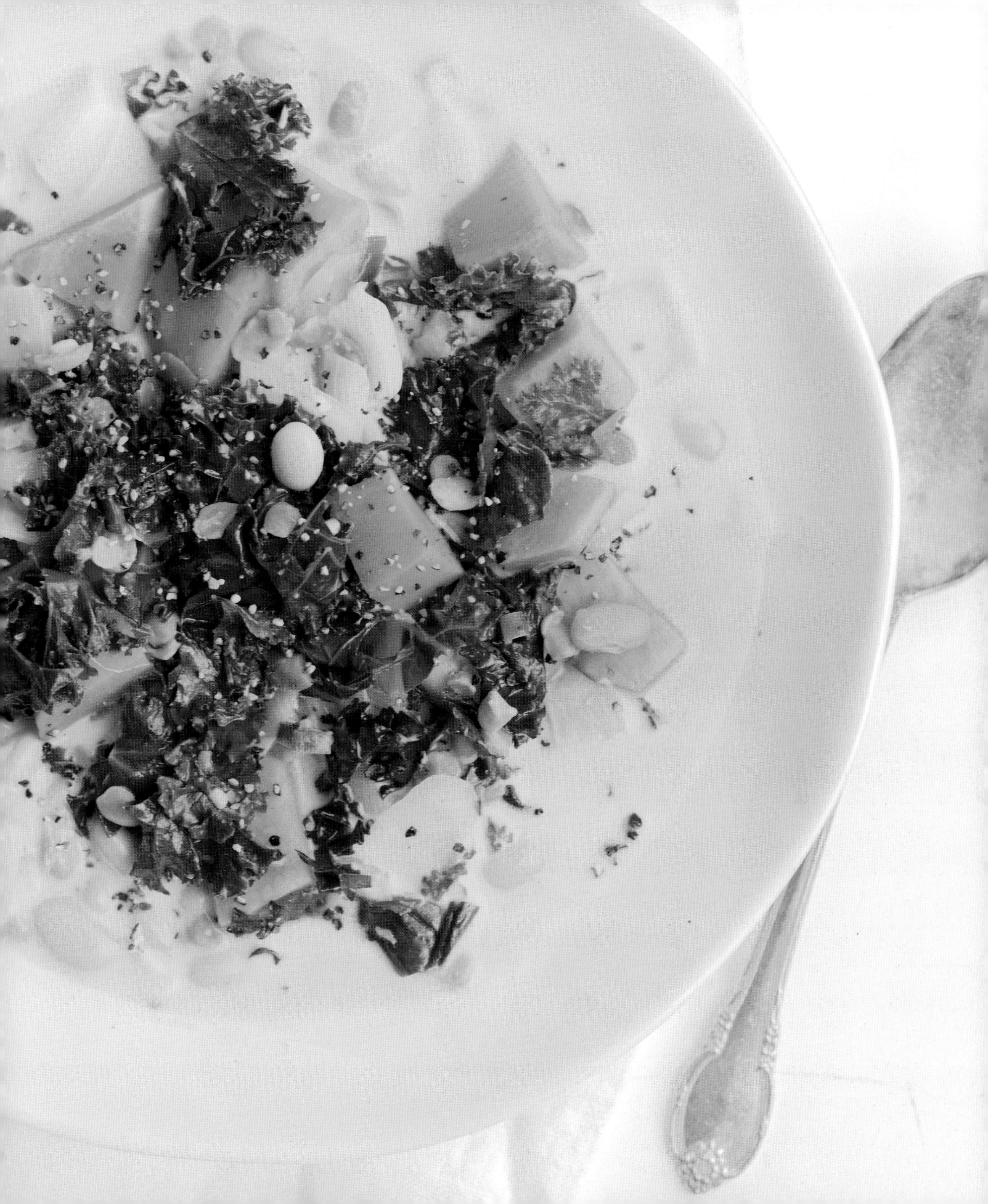

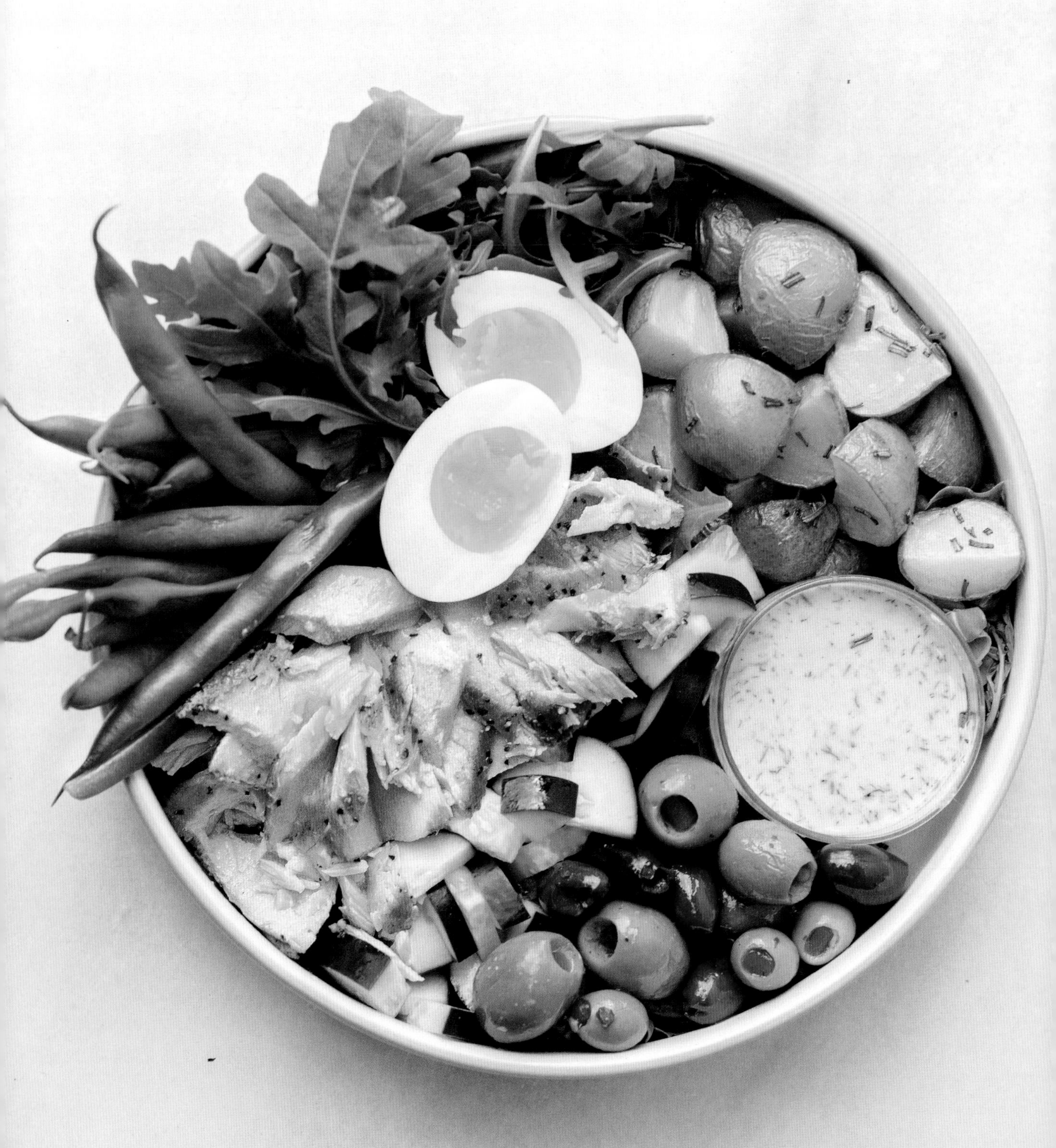

salmon niçoise salad

Get your omega-3 boost in this Niçoise salad with a salmon twist. Olives add to the heart-healthy fat content while the vegetable assortment adds fiber and a refreshing crunch to every bite. Even the dressing boasts an additional 3 grams of protein per serving from the secret creamy weapon, tahini! All that fiber, fat, and protein work together to make a delicious and blood sugar–balancing meal.

gluten-free | high fiber | protein packed | yield: 1 serving

salad

4 oz (113 g) fresh salmon fillets

Cooking oil spray, as needed

1 tsp olive oil

Sea salt, as needed

Black pepper, as needed

2 cups (60 g) arugula

⅛ cup (17 g) assorted olives

½ cup (60 g) coarsely chopped cucumber

1 large hard-boiled egg

½ cup (65 g) quartered baby potatoes

2 tsp (2 g) dried rosemary

2½ oz (71 g) fresh green beans

dressing

1 tbsp (15 g) tahini

½ tbsp (8 g) Dijon mustard

1 tbsp (15 ml) fresh lemon juice

3 tbsp (45 ml) water

½ tsp dried dill

Sea salt, as needed

Black pepper, as needed

Preheat the oven to 400°F (204°C). Line a large baking sheet with parchment paper.

Bring a large pot of water to a boil over high heat.

To make the salad, heat a medium skillet over medium-high heat. Spray the salmon with the cooking oil spray and drizzle the oil on top. Place it in the skillet and cook for 2 to 3 minutes on each side (depending how thick the fillet is), until the outside is an opaque pink color and just barely starts to brown. Season the salmon with the salt and black pepper.

On a serving plate, arrange a bed of arugula. On the arugula, arrange the olives, cucumber, egg, and salmon. Set the plate aside.

Place the potatoes in a medium bowl. Add the rosemary and toss to coat the potatoes. Transfer them to the prepared baking sheet and bake them for 20 to 25 minutes, or until the potatoes are brown and crispy on the outside.

While the potatoes are roasting, prepare a large bowl of ice water. Add the green beans to the boiling water and cook them for 2 minutes. Quickly transfer the green beans to the bowl of ice water. Once they have cooled, add the green beans to the salad.

To make the dressing, mix together the tahini, mustard, lemon juice, water, dill, sea salt, and black pepper in a medium jar.

Add the potatoes to the salad, toss the salad with the dressing, and serve.

STORAGE: Serve the salad immediately, as it does not keep well.

Estimated Nutrition Facts per Serving: 471 calories; 31 g carbs; 7 g fiber; 6 g sugar; 37 g protein; 23 g fat (4 g saturated fat); 555 mg sodium

cheeseburger wedge salad

This salad takes everything you love about a juicy cheeseburger and serves it up in salad form! The crispy crunch of the lettuce combined with your favorite cheeseburger toppings and a homemade "ketchup dressing" is the perfect easy lunch or dinner option. And the lower carbohydrate content makes it a much more blood sugar–friendly option than a traditional cheeseburger.

gluten-free | high fiber | protein packed | yield: 4 servings

salad

1 lb (454 g) lean ground beef

2 medium heads romaine lettuce, rinsed, dried, and sliced in half lengthwise

½ cup (60 g) shredded Cheddar cheese

½ cup (80 g) coarsely chopped tomatoes

⅓ cup (50 g) finely chopped red onion

1 small dill pickle, finely chopped (optional)

dressing

2 oz (57 g) no-salt-added tomato paste

2 tbsp (30 ml) apple cider vinegar

2 tbsp (30 ml) water

1 tbsp (15 ml) honey

¼ tsp sea salt

½ tsp onion powder

¼ tsp garlic powder

To make the salad, heat a large skillet over medium-high heat. Once the skillet is hot, add the beef and cook it for 9 to 10 minutes, until it is brown and cooked though.

Meanwhile, place a ½ head of romaine lettuce on each of four plates. Divide the beef evenly on top of each of the romaine halves. Then top each with the Cheddar cheese, tomatoes, onion, and pickle (if using).

To make the dressing, combine the tomato paste, vinegar, water, honey, sea salt, onion powder, and garlic powder in a small mason jar, secure the lid on top, and shake the jar thoroughly until everything is combined. Drizzle the dressing evenly over each salad and serve.

STORAGE: Eat this salad immediately, as it does not keep well.

Estimated Nutrition Facts per Serving without Toppings: 320 calories; 19 g carbs; 8 g fiber; 11 g sugar (4 g added sugar); 32 g protein; 14 g fat (6 g saturated fat); 341 mg sodium

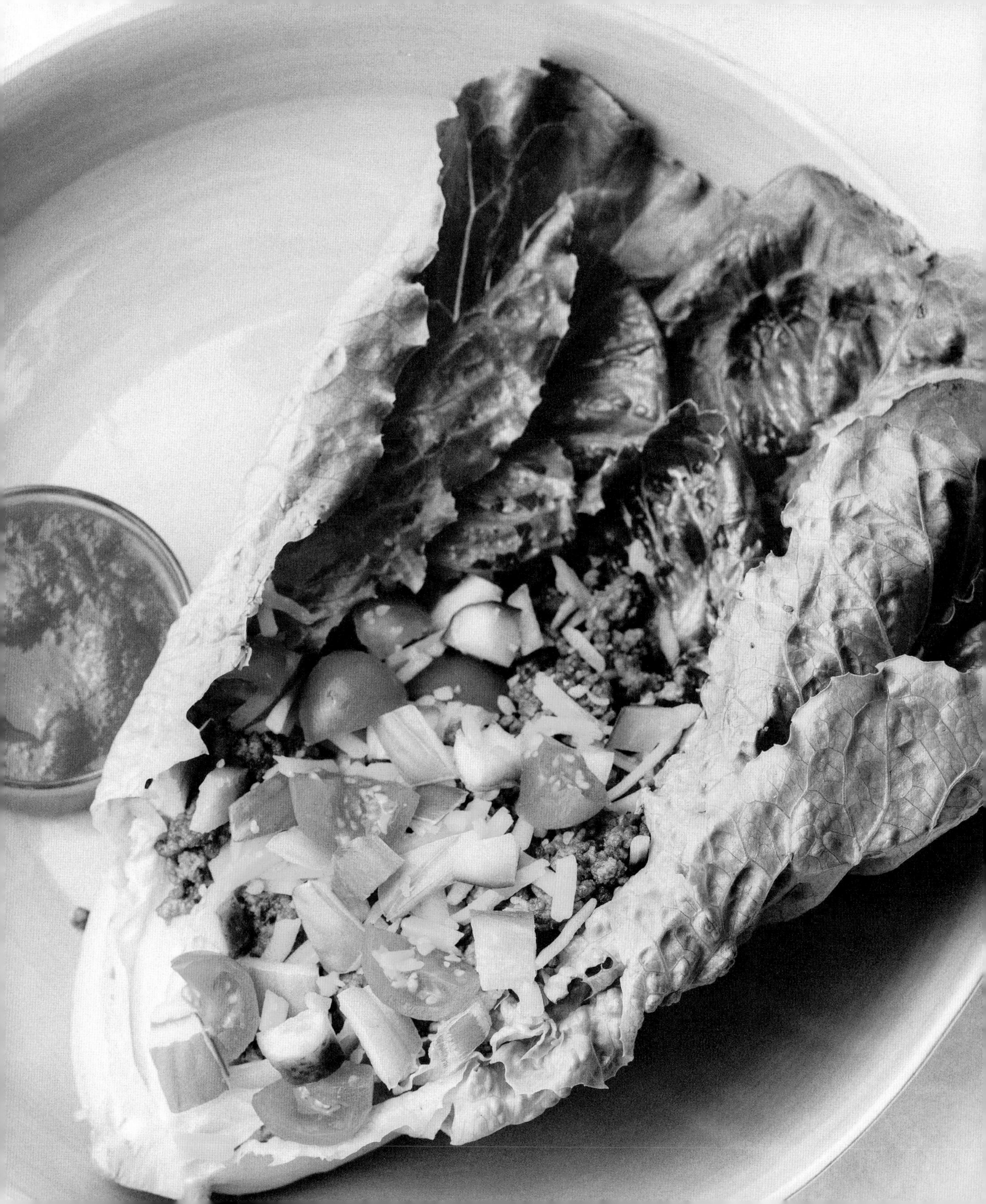

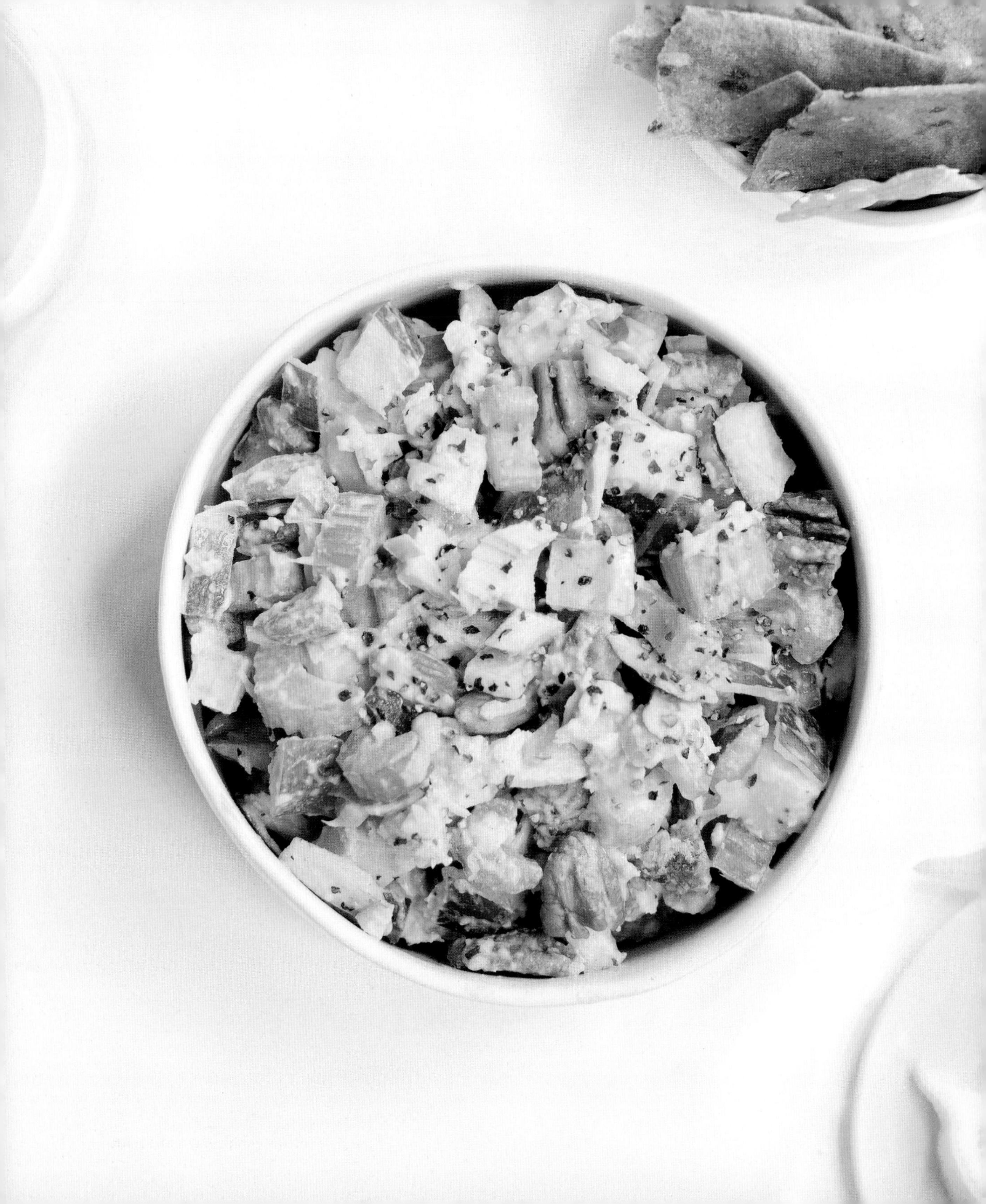

crunchy pecan tuna salad

Boring tuna salad just got a little more fiber-rich and flavorful! Instead of drowning tuna in lots of mayo, I use just a bit of it and mix in mashed white beans for a creamy, nutritious twist. This option lowers the saturated fat while boosting the fiber and protein, which makes blood sugars happy. I also added some fruits, veggies, and pecans to make this tuna salad juicy, crunchy, and perfectly balanced between tart and sweet.

gluten-free | high fiber | no added sugar | sodium aware | yield: 1 serving

½ medium apple, finely chopped

2 medium ribs celery, finely chopped

¼ large red onion, finely chopped

2 tbsp (16 g) coarsely chopped pecans

¼ cup (46 g) canned navy beans, drained, rinsed, and mashed

2 oz (57 g) canned tuna packed in water, drained and rinsed

1 tbsp (14 g) mayonnaise (see Tip)

½ tbsp (8 g) Dijon mustard

1 tbsp (15 ml) fresh lemon juice

Black pepper, as needed

In a large bowl, combine the apple, celery, onion, pecans, beans, and tuna.

In a small bowl, mix together the mayonnaise, mustard, lemon juice, and black pepper. Add the mayonnaise mixture to the tuna mixture and stir until the tuna salad is evenly combined.

Serve the tuna salad immediately, or refrigerate the tuna salad for 2 to 3 hours or overnight to chill it and allow the flavors to meld.

STORAGE: Store the tuna salad in a sealed container in the refrigerator for up to 3 days.

TIP: If you like your tuna salad with a kick, you can substitute 1½ tablespoons (21 g) of chipotle mayonnaise for the mayonnaise and Dijon mustard.

Estimated Nutrition Facts per Serving: 197 calories; 16 g carbs; 5 g fiber; 7 g sugar; 11 g protein; 11 g fat (1 g saturated fat); 179 mg sodium

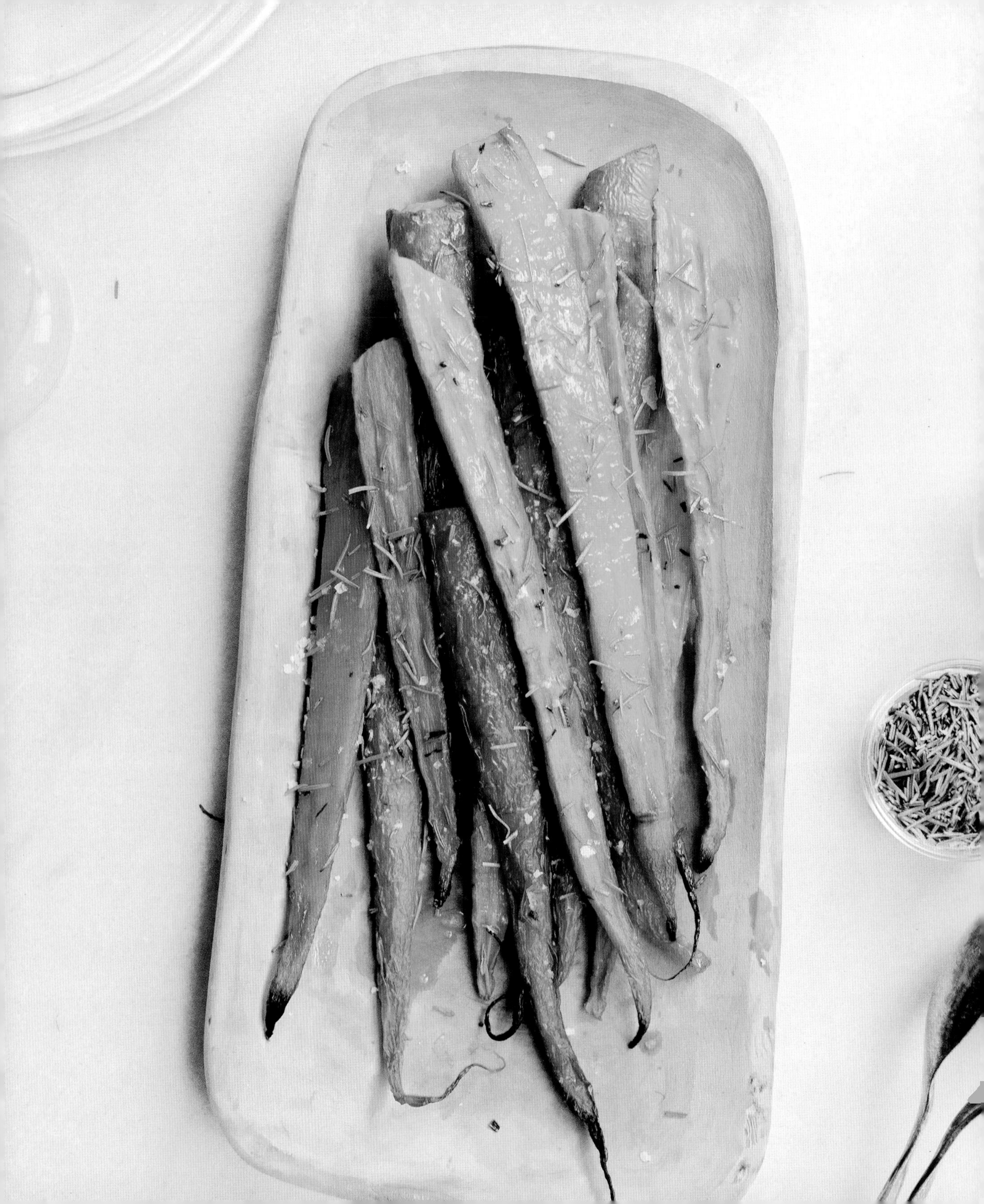

flavorful veggies

NUTRITIOUS SIDE DISHES YOU'LL ACTUALLY WANT TO EAT

It's no secret that a diet rich in vegetables is good for you. Eating a variety of vegetables throughout the day each day is associated with reduced risk and improved symptoms of many chronic illnesses, including diabetes. Veggies help make blood sugars easier to manage because of their fiber and protein content—yes, vegetables have protein too! And don't forget, they're good for everyone because of all those vitamins, minerals, and antioxidants.

But many people with diabetes don't eat enough vegetables. I've found that this is usually because people don't know how to prepare vegetables in healthy and tasty ways. I get it—I don't like bland and boring steamed veggies either. Thankfully, all of the recipes in the next few pages are not only blood sugar–friendly but are also full of flavor that will leave you wanting more!

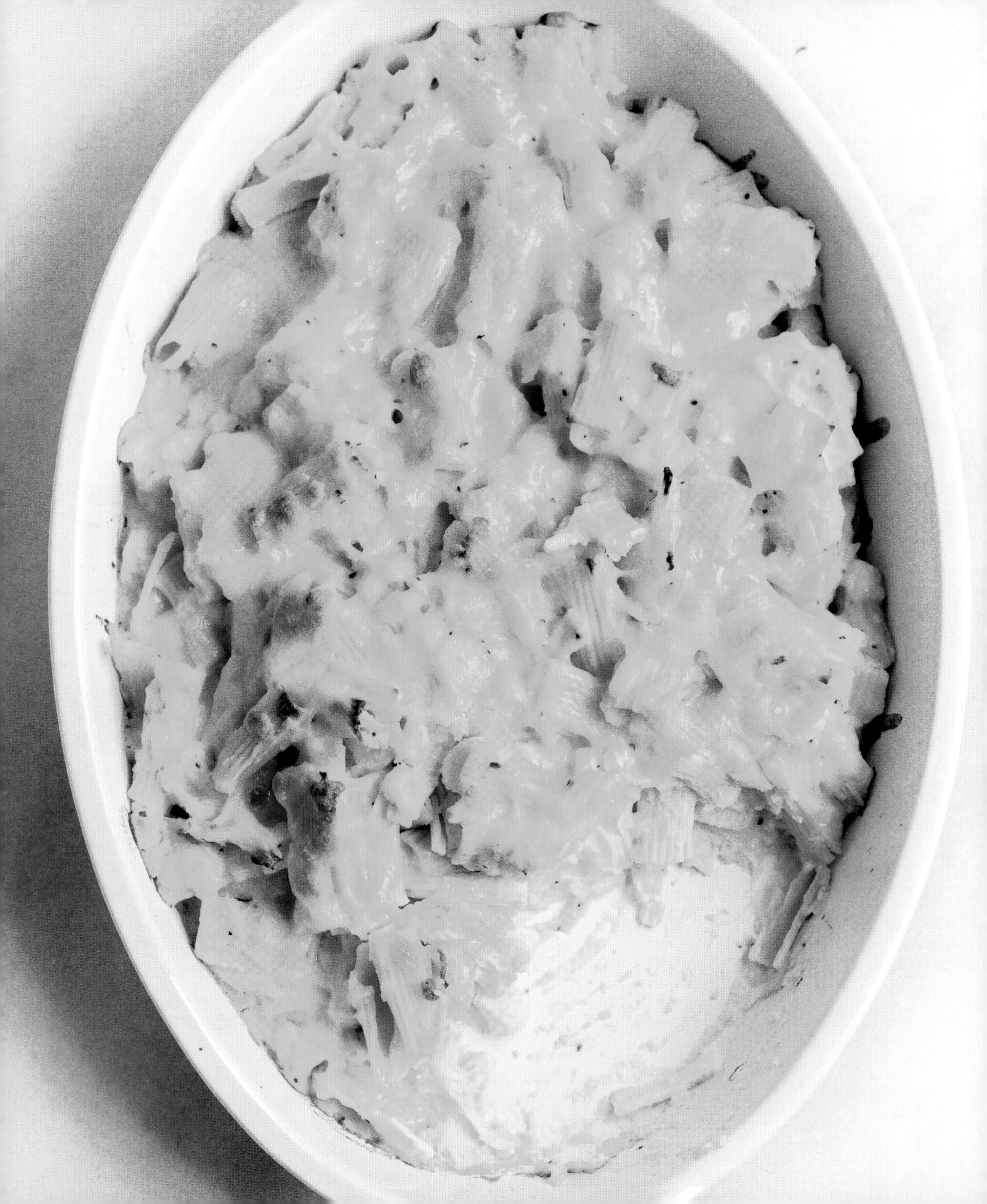

cauliflower and butternut squash mac and cheese

Mac and cheese gets a veggie boost in this baked casserole classic. Not only do the cauliflower and butternut squash add more fiber and lower the saturated fat content of traditional mac and cheese but they also provide a creamy and flavorful sauce that complements the Cheddar cheese. This recipe also uses chickpea pasta, which is higher in protein and lower in carbohydrates than traditional pasta options.

gluten-free | high fiber | no added sugar | protein packed | yield: 4 servings

1 lb (454 g) chickpea pasta (any shape)

1 lb (454 g) cauliflower florets

1 (1-lb [454-g]) butternut squash, peeled and cubed

1 tsp garlic powder

1 cup (240 ml) low-sodium vegetable broth

Sea salt, as needed

Black pepper, as needed

1 cup (120 g) shredded Cheddar cheese, divided

Preheat the oven to 400°F (204°C).

Bring two large pots of water to a boil over high heat.

Add the pasta to one pot of water and the cauliflower and butternut squash to the other. Cook the pasta according to the package directions and boil the vegetables for 10 to 12 minutes, until they are fork-tender.

Drain the pasta and transfer it to a large baking dish.

Drain the cauliflower and squash and transfer them to a high-power blender. Add the garlic powder, broth, sea salt, black pepper, and ¾ cup (90 g) of the Cheddar cheese. Blend until the sauce is smooth and creamy.

Pour the cheese sauce over the pasta and stir it to evenly distribute it throughout the pasta. Sprinkle the remaining ¼ cup (30 g) of Cheddar cheese over the top of the pasta. Bake the mac and cheese for 25 minutes, or until the cheese is melted and lightly browned.

STORAGE: Store the mac and cheese in an airtight container in the refrigerator for up to 5 days.

Estimated Nutrition Facts per Serving: 388 calories; 53 g carbs; 13 g fiber; 10 g sugar; 25 g protein; 13 g fat (5 g saturated fat); 315 mg sodium

classic oven-roasted carrots

Carrots offer a rich, naturally sweet flavor that is best captured by roasting. Their sweetness is the perfect addition to an easy weeknight meal or a fancier special occasion. Their fiber and antioxidant content also make them a great blood sugar–friendly veggie.

gluten-free | high fiber | no added sugar | vegan | yield: 4 servings

1½ lbs (680 g) large carrots, trimmed and washed

Avocado oil spray, as needed

¼ tsp sea salt

1 tbsp (3 g) dried rosemary

Preheat the oven to 400°F (204°C). Line a large baking sheet with parchment paper.

Arrange the carrots on the prepared baking sheet, making sure there is at least ½ inch (13 mm) between each of them.

Generously spray the carrots with the avocado oil spray, and then sprinkle them with the sea salt and rosemary. Roast the carrots for 15 minutes, or until they are fork-tender.

STORAGE: Store the carrots in an airtight container in the refrigerator for up to 7 days.

Estimated Nutrition Facts per Serving: 72 calories; 17 g carbs; 5 g fiber; 8 g sugar; 2 g protein; 1 g fat; 263 mg sodium

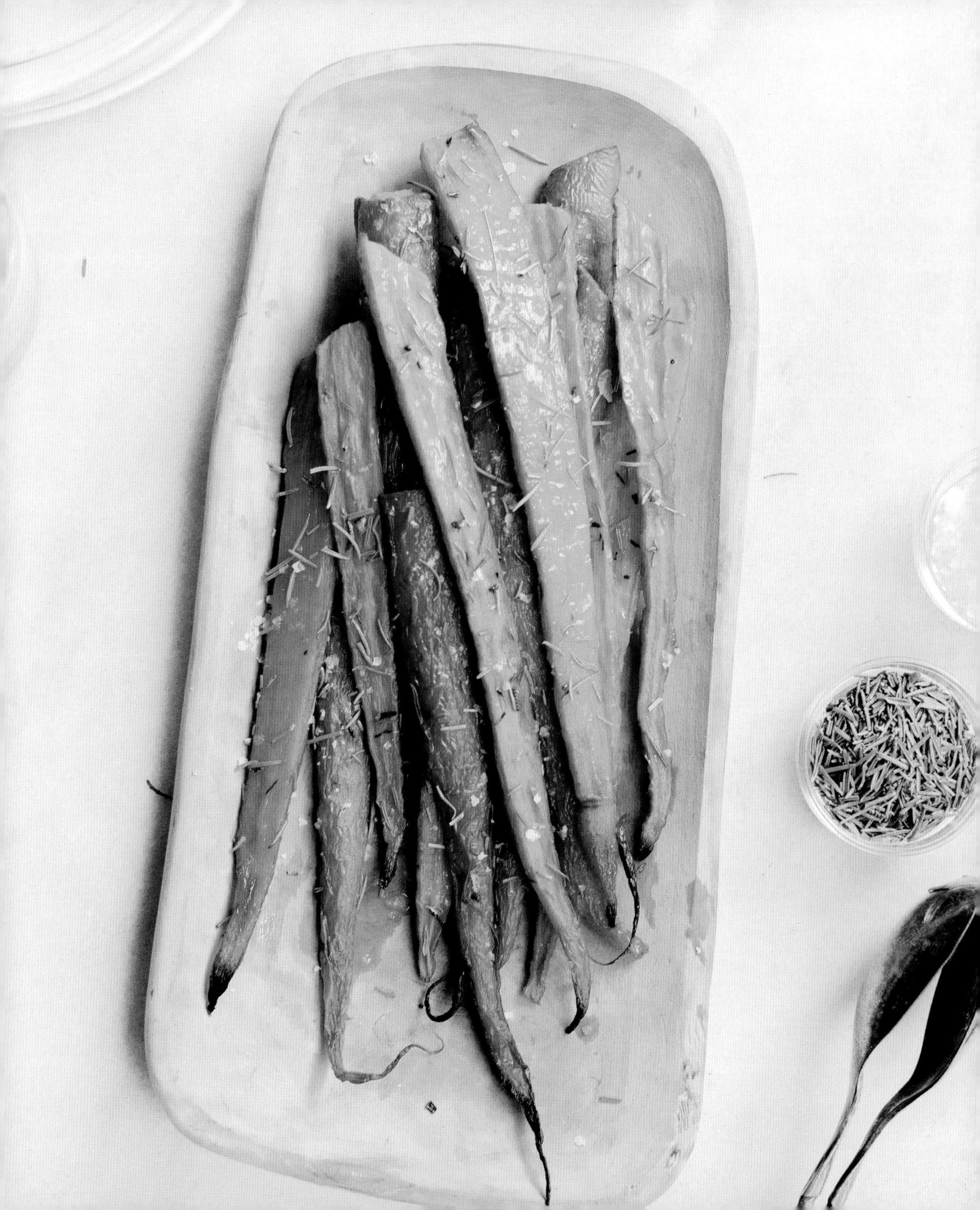

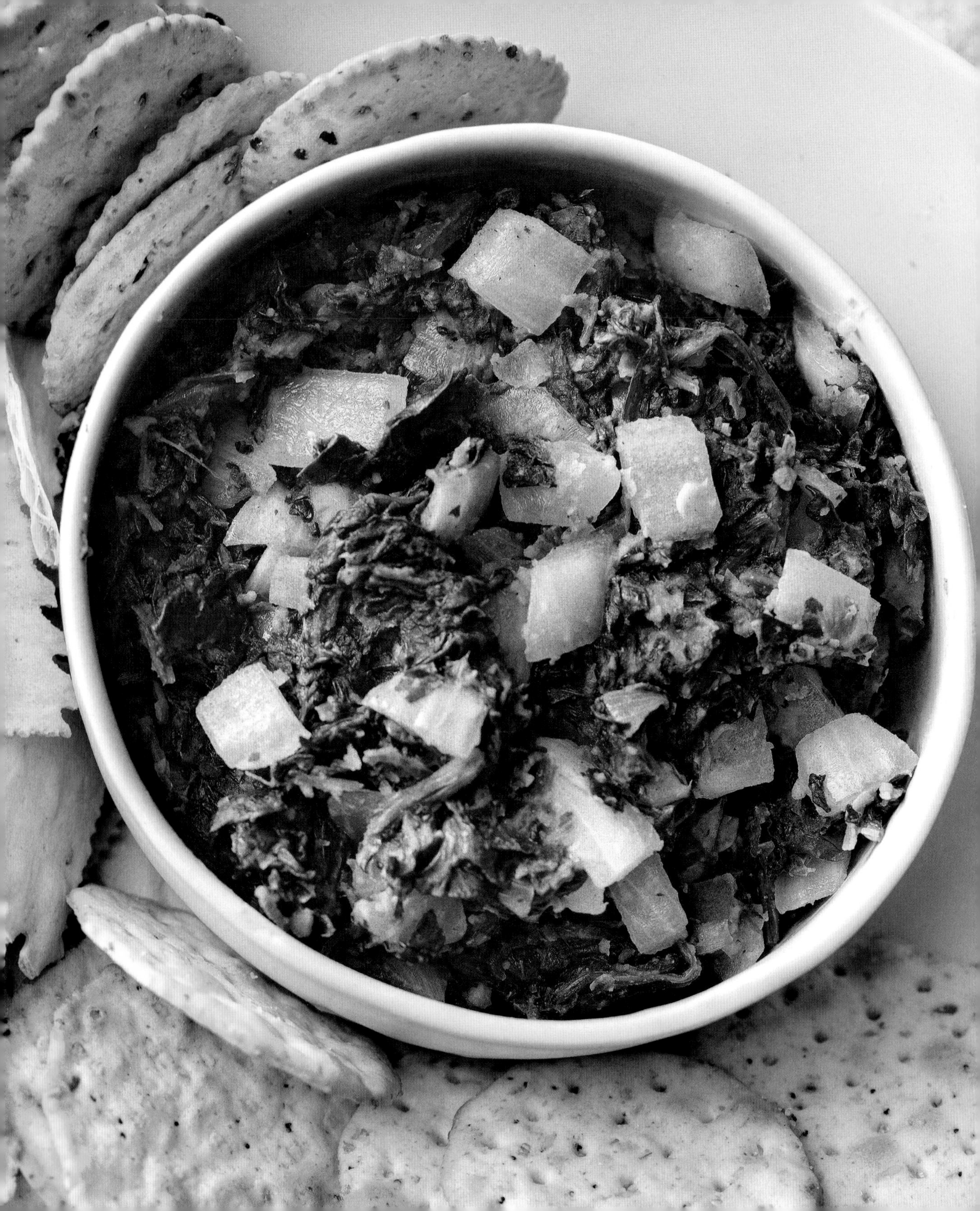

garlic creamed spinach

Creamed spinach gets a high-fiber, low-fat, high-protein makeover with white beans. All of these changes make this dish the perfect blood sugar–friendly side dish. One serving has about a third of your daily recommended intake of fiber! The dish comes together in fewer than 15 minutes and makes a great dip as well as a side dish.

gluten-free | high fiber | no added sugar | sodium aware | vegan | yield: 4 servings

2 tsp (10 ml) olive oil

2 cloves garlic, coarsely chopped

1 medium onion, finely chopped

1 lb (454 g) frozen spinach, thawed

1 (15-oz [425-g]) can white beans of choice, undrained

Sea salt, as needed

Black pepper, as needed

Heat the oil in a large skillet over medium heat. Add the garlic and onion and sauté them for about 5 minutes, until they are brown and fragrant.

Meanwhile, drain the spinach in a colander to remove as much excess water as possible. Add the spinach to the skillet.

In a food processor or blender, purée the white beans and their liquid until they are thick and creamy. Stir the white bean purée into the spinach mixture.

Let the creamed spinach cook for 5 minutes, until it is warmed through. Season it with the sea salt and black pepper and serve.

STORAGE: Store the spinach in an airtight container in the refrigerator for up to 5 days.

Estimated Nutrition Facts per Serving: 168 calories; 28 g carbs; 9 g fiber; 6 g sugar; 9 g protein; 2 g fat; 216 mg sodium

lean green avocado mashed potatoes

These lightened-up mashed potatoes are packed with fiber from the potato skins, cauliflower, and avocado. They are much kinder to blood sugars than traditional mashed potatoes, and I think they taste a hundred times more delicious too! The avocado also adds a boost of heart-healthy fat and creaminess without overpowering the dish.

gluten-free | high fiber | no added sugar | sodium aware | vegan | yield: 4 servings

2 large russet potatoes, chopped

1 large head cauliflower, cut into 1-inch (2.5-cm) florets

2 medium leeks, washed and coarsely chopped

2 tsp (10 ml) olive oil

1 tbsp (3 g) dried rosemary

1 tbsp (3 g) dried thyme

2 cloves garlic

1 medium avocado, peeled and pitted

2 tbsp (8 g) finely chopped fresh chives

Preheat the oven to 400°F (204°C).

Spread out the potatoes, cauliflower, and leeks on a large baking sheet. Drizzle the vegetables with the oil, then sprinkle them with the rosemary and thyme. Add the garlic to the baking sheet. Bake the vegetables for about 30 minutes, until the potatoes are fork-tender.

Transfer the vegetables to a food processor and add the avocado. Process the mixture to the desired consistency.

Top the mashed potatoes with the chives and serve.

STORAGE: Store the mashed potatoes in an airtight container in the refrigerator for up to 5 days.

Estimated Nutrition Facts per Serving: 248 calories; 37 g carbs; 9 g fiber; 6 g sugar; 7 g protein; 10 g fat (2 g saturated fat); 69 mg sodium

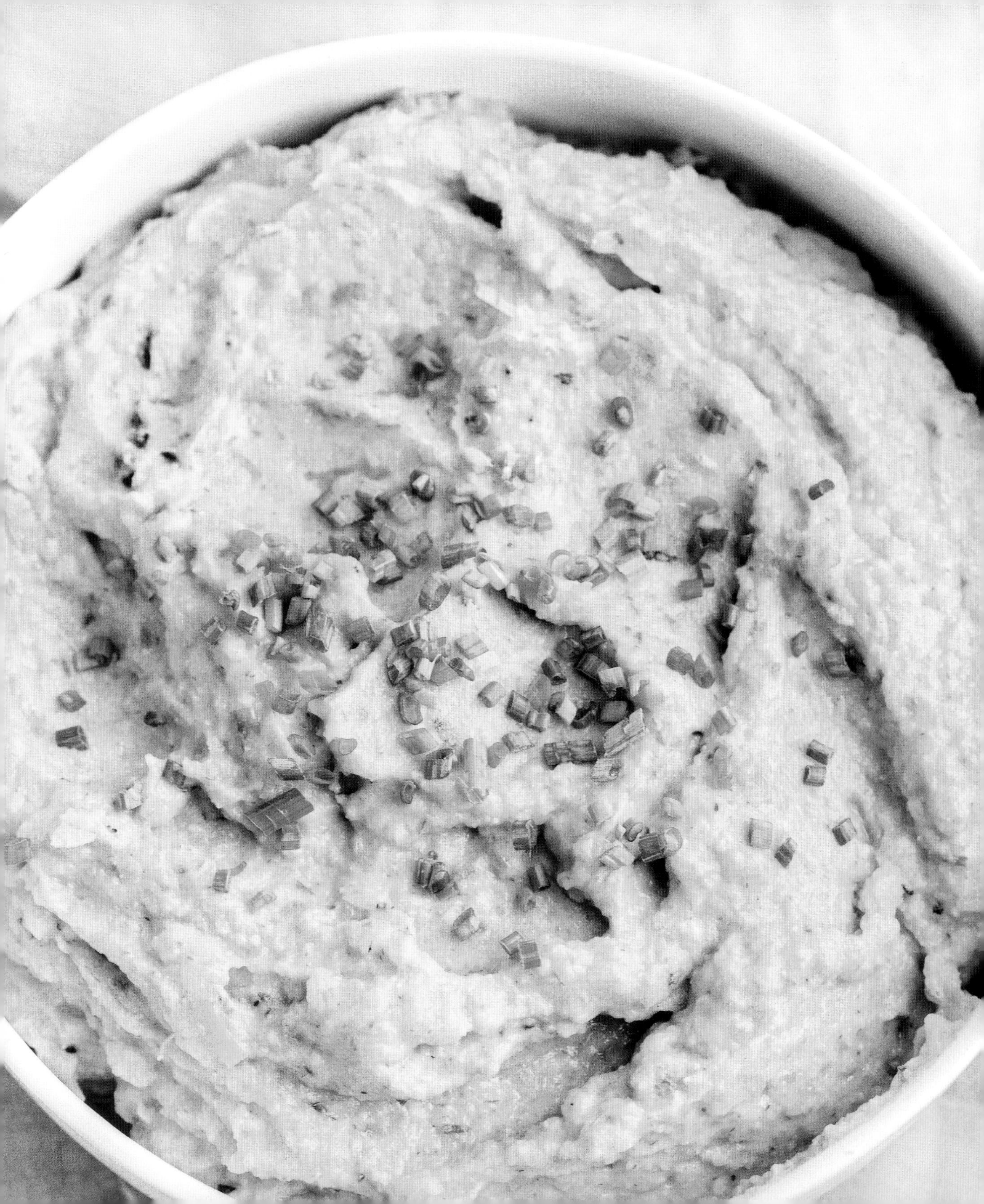

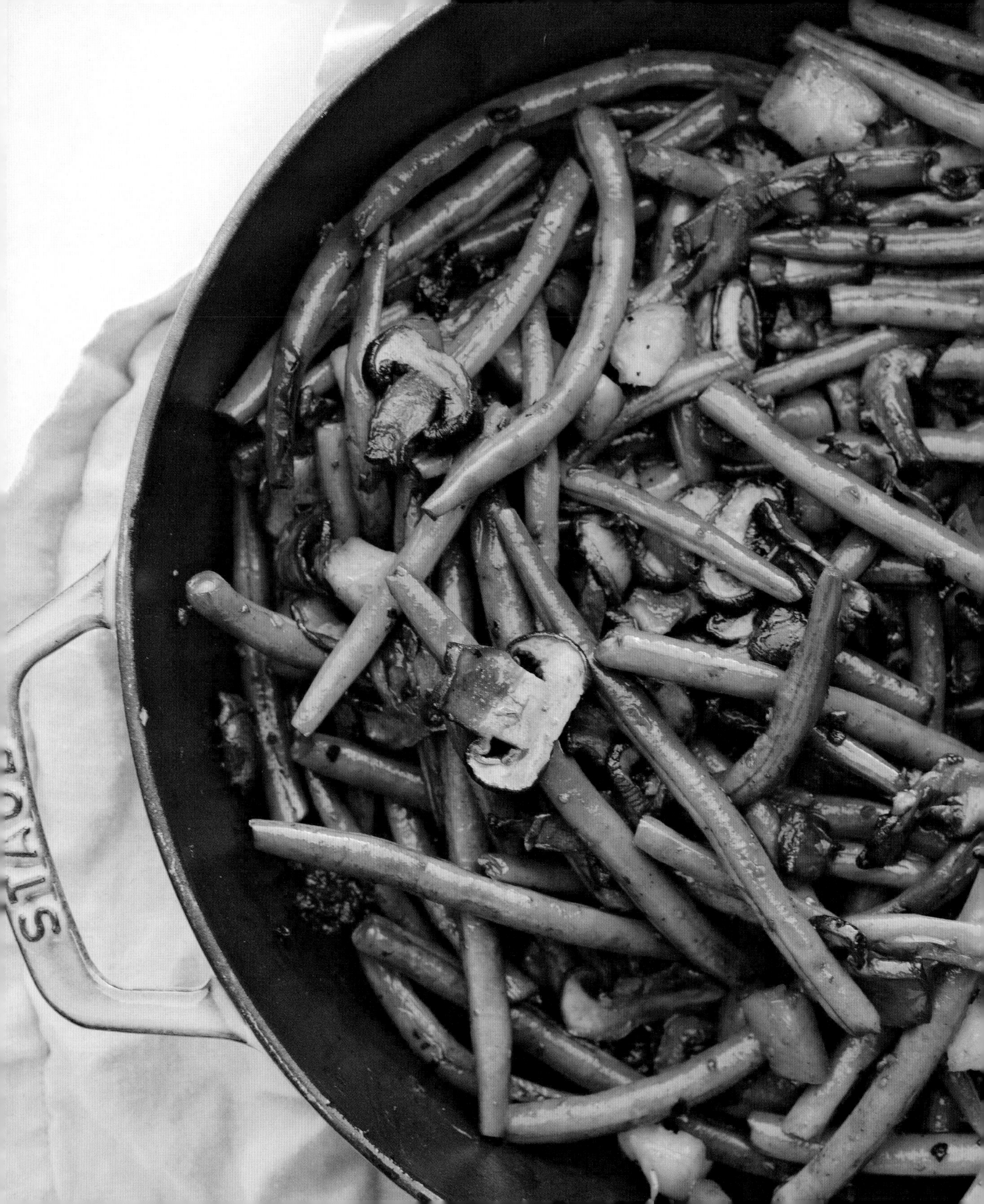
STAUB

teriyaki green beans

Move aside, takeout! These sweet and savory green beans get their sweetness from fresh pineapple, which also adds a boost of fiber. This dish packs in even more veggies with crispy mushrooms, which add an umami flavor and can be either roasted or stir-fried, depending on how much time you have to cook. This satisfying high-protein side comes together even faster than ordering takeout and will leave your blood sugars steady, unlike some traditional takeout options.

gluten-free | high fiber | no added sugar | vegan | yield: 4 servings

10 oz (283 g) button mushrooms, thinly sliced

1 tbsp (15 ml) sesame oil, divided

2 tbsp (30 ml) low-sodium tamari, divided

½ tsp smoked paprika

2 cloves garlic, minced

1 lb (454 g) fresh green beans, trimmed and washed

1 cup (165 g) finely chopped fresh pineapple

In a large bowl, combine the mushrooms with ½ tablespoon (8 ml) of the oil, 1½ tablespoons (23 ml) of the tamari, and the smoked paprika. Let the mushrooms rest for 10 minutes to allow them to absorb the marinade.

If you will be roasting the mushrooms, preheat the oven to 400°F (204°C) while the mushrooms marinate. Line a large baking sheet with parchment paper.

Spread out the mushrooms on the prepared baking sheet. Roast them for 20 minutes, or until they are very crispy.

Alternatively, if you will be stir-frying the mushrooms, heat a small skillet over medium heat. Add the mushrooms and stir-fry them for about 5 minutes, until they are tender. Note that this cooking method will yield mushrooms that are less crispy than roasting, but they will still be delicious.

Meanwhile, heat the remaining ½ tablespoon (8 ml) of oil in a large skillet over medium-high heat. Add the garlic and cook it for 2 minutes, or until it is brown and fragrant. Add the green beans and pineapple. Cook the mixture for 10 minutes, until the green beans are bright green and starting to soften. Add the crispy mushrooms to the skillet. Stir to combine, then serve.

STORAGE: Store the green beans in an airtight container in the refrigerator for up to 5 days.

Estimated Nutrition Facts per Serving: 106 calories; 17 g carbs; 5 g fiber; 9 g sugar; 6 g protein; 3 g fat (<1g saturated fat); 257 mg sodium

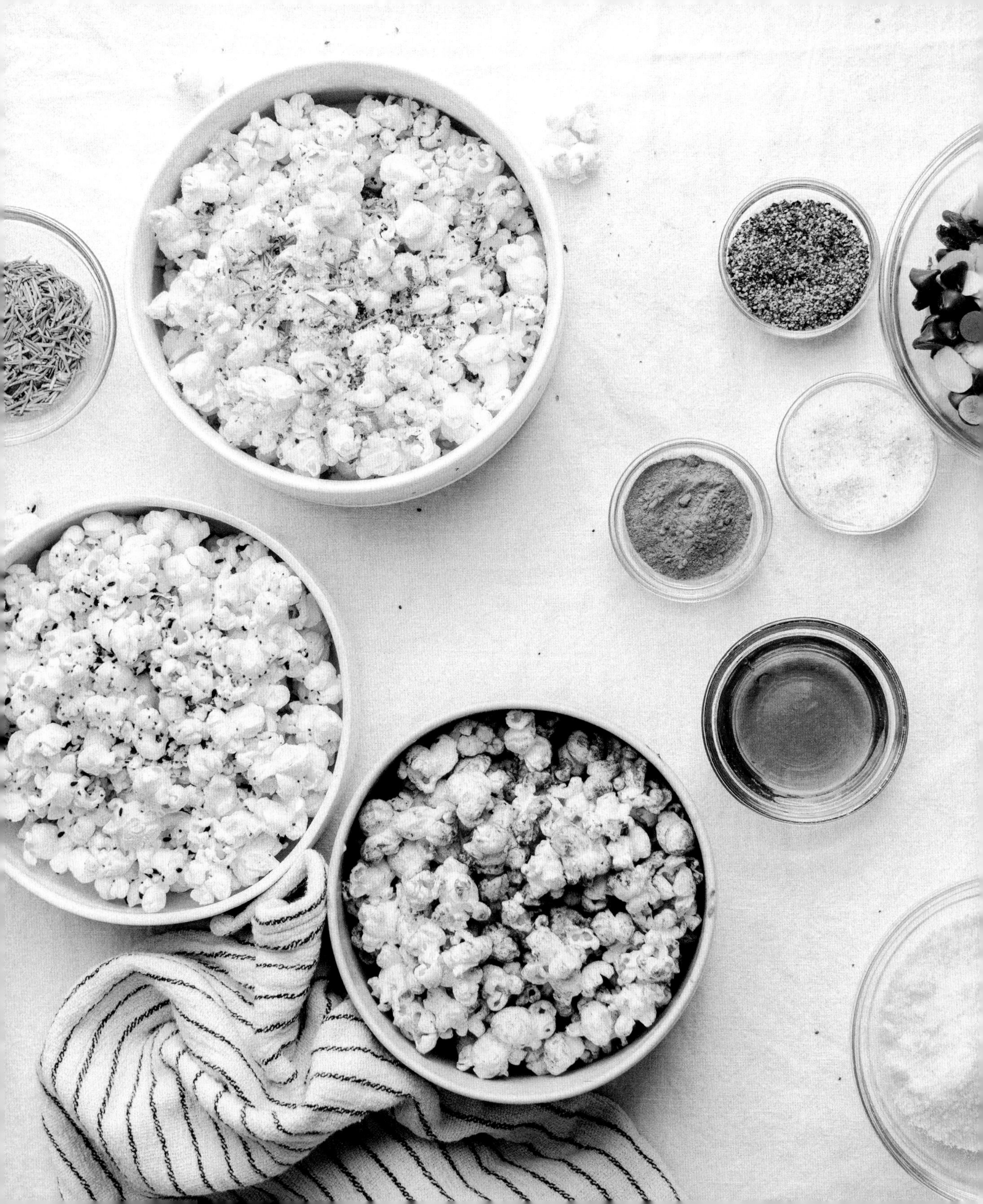

wholesome snacks

BALANCED BITES TO GET YOU FROM ONE MEAL TO THE NEXT

We eat snacks for many reasons: We're hungry, we need fuel, we are about to work out, we are bored. But the primary reason for a snack is that we need something to get us from one meal to the next. Snacks keep us full and energized—or at least keep our stomachs from growling! Whether it's midmorning, late afternoon, or bedtime, everyone enjoys a good snack, especially if it's tasty and satisfying.

To truly understand why we eat snacks, though, we need to do a brief review of our macro nutrients: carbohydrates, protein, and fat. These three things are the only things that provide calories to our bodies. (The exception is alcohol, which also provides calories but isn't considered a nutrient.) They each serve different functions in our bodies and are absorbed at different speeds. Carbohydrates leave our stomachs and get absorbed and digested faster than protein and fat do, to give us quick energy. If eaten by themselves, they can raise blood sugars quicker than desired.

Protein and fat, on the other hand, help keep us energized over longer periods of time. They slow down the absorption of carbohydrates and provide a slower, steadier supply of energy. So the "ideal" snack would combine the quick energy of carbohydrates and sustained satiety of fat and protein. This is why an apple by itself (carbohydrate) only keeps you full for an hour, but an apple with peanut butter (which adds protein and fat) keeps you full longer. Carbohydrates plus protein and fat equals sustained energy, fullness, and stable blood sugars.

There are so many great carb-protein-fat combinations to pick from:

- Low-Sugar Blueberry Muffins (page 111)
- An apple slathered with peanut butter
- No-Bake Coconut and Cashew Energy Bars (page 112)
- Carrots and hummus
- Avocado toast
- Cheese and crackers
- Homemade Sun-Dried Tomato Salsa (page 119) with veggies

All of these ideas make the "ideal" snack for someone with diabetes because they offer that perfect balance of carbs and protein or fat. My No-Bake Coconut and Cashew Energy Bars (page 112) are loaded with better-for-you fats and protein and can be made ahead for a quick blood sugar–balancing snack. And the Homemade Sun-Dried Tomato Salsa (page 119) can be paired with whole-grain crackers, chips, or veggies for an afternoon pick-me-up filled with fiber and plant-based fats.

These wholesome and blood sugar–balancing snack recipes are the perfect way to help you get from one meal to the next with a satisfied tummy and a steady supply of energy.

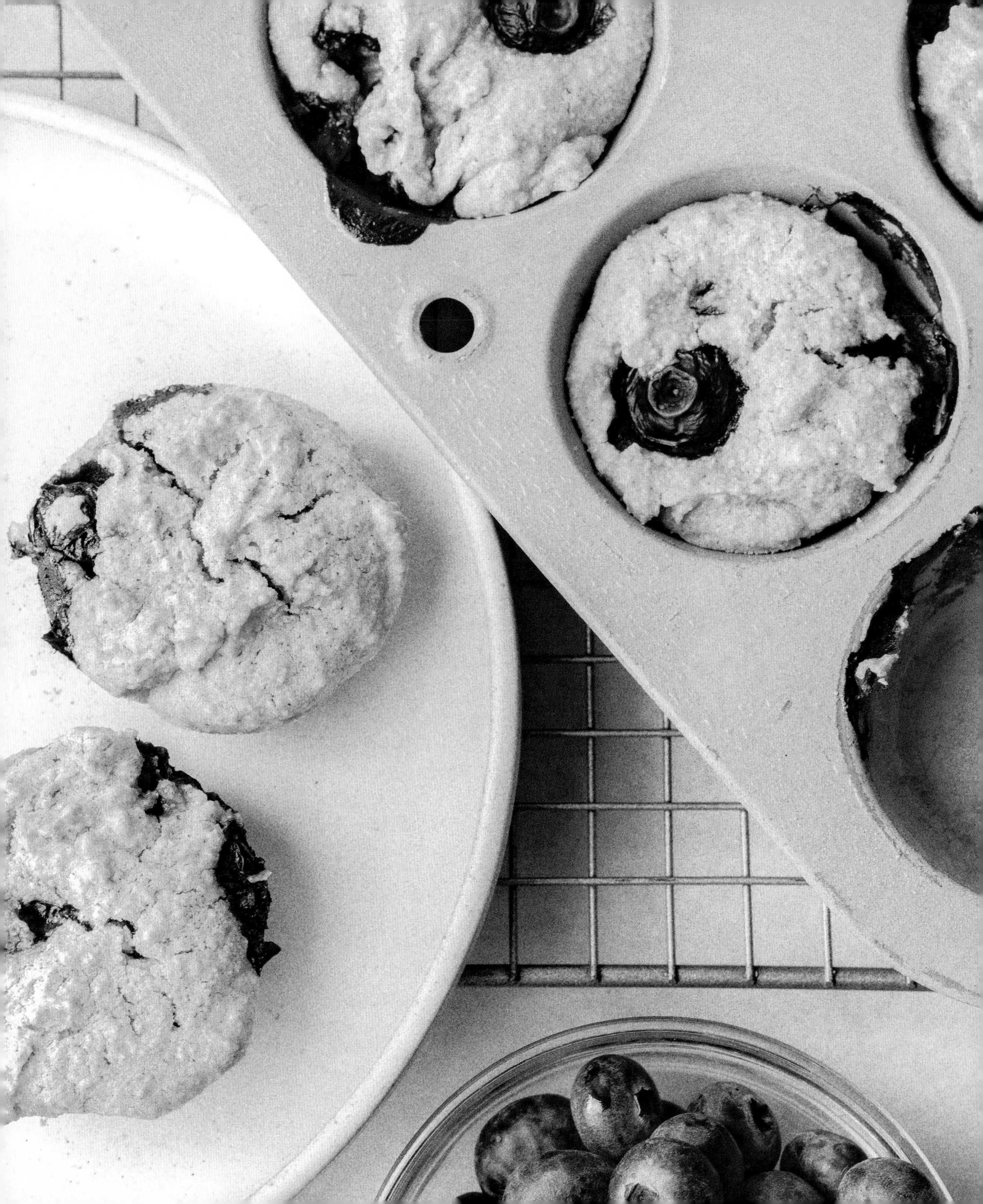

low-sugar blueberry muffins

These muffins are an easy low-sugar snack you can whip up in no time. They're loaded with plant-based fat and a good dose of protein. These muffins impact blood sugars less than traditional muffins. And I love adding blueberries to dishes—they're a quality source of many nutrients, including vitamin C, fiber, and manganese.

gluten-free | sodium aware | yield: 12 muffins

2 large eggs

1½ cups (144 g) almond flour

1 cup (80 g) gluten-free rolled oats

½ cup (120 ml) pure maple syrup

½ cup (120 ml) avocado oil

1 tsp baking powder

1 tsp ground cinnamon

½ tsp pure vanilla extract

½ tsp pure almond extract

1 cup (150 g) fresh or frozen blueberries

Preheat the oven to 350°F (177°C). Line a 12-well muffin pan with paper liners or spray the wells with cooking oil spray.

In a blender, combine the eggs, almond flour, oats, maple syrup, oil, baking powder, cinnamon, vanilla, and almond extract. Blend the ingredients on high for 20 to 30 seconds, until the mixture is homogeneous.

Transfer the batter to a large bowl and gently stir in the blueberries.

Divide the batter evenly among the muffin wells. Bake the muffins for 20 to 25 minutes, until a toothpick inserted in the middle comes out clean.

Let the muffins rest for 5 minutes, then transfer them to a cooling rack.

STORAGE: Store the muffins in a sealed container in the refrigerator for up to 1 week, or freeze them for up to 6 months.

Estimated Nutrition Facts per Serving: 240 calories; 19 g carbs; 3 g fiber; 10 g sugar; 5 g protein; 18 g fat (2 g saturated fat); 19 mg sodium

no-bake coconut and cashew energy bars

It doesn't get much easier than four ingredients and no baking! These energy bars are not only simple but they're also a great source of plant-based fat and great for on-the-go snacking. The combo of fat, fiber, and protein makes them the perfect energy bars for people with diabetes.

gluten-free | low carb | sodium aware | vegan | yield: 12 energy bars

1 cup (110 g) raw cashews

1 cup (80 g) unsweetened shredded coconut

½ cup (120 g) unsweetened nut butter of choice

2 tbsp (30 ml) pure maple syrup

Line an 8 x 8–inch (20 x 20–cm) baking pan with parchment paper.

In a large food processor, combine the cashews and coconut. Pulse them for 15 to 20 seconds to form a powder.

Add the nut butter and maple syrup and process until a doughy paste is formed, scraping down the sides if needed.

Spread the dough into the prepared baking pan. Cover the dough with another sheet of parchment paper and press it flat.

Freeze the dough for 1 hour. Cut the dough into bars.

STORAGE: Eat these bars immediately or store them in the refrigerator for up to 2 weeks, or freeze them for up to 6 months.

Estimated Nutrition Facts per Serving: 169 calories; 10 g carbs; 2 g fiber; 3 g sugar; 4 g protein; 14 g fat (6 g saturated fat); 6 mg sodium

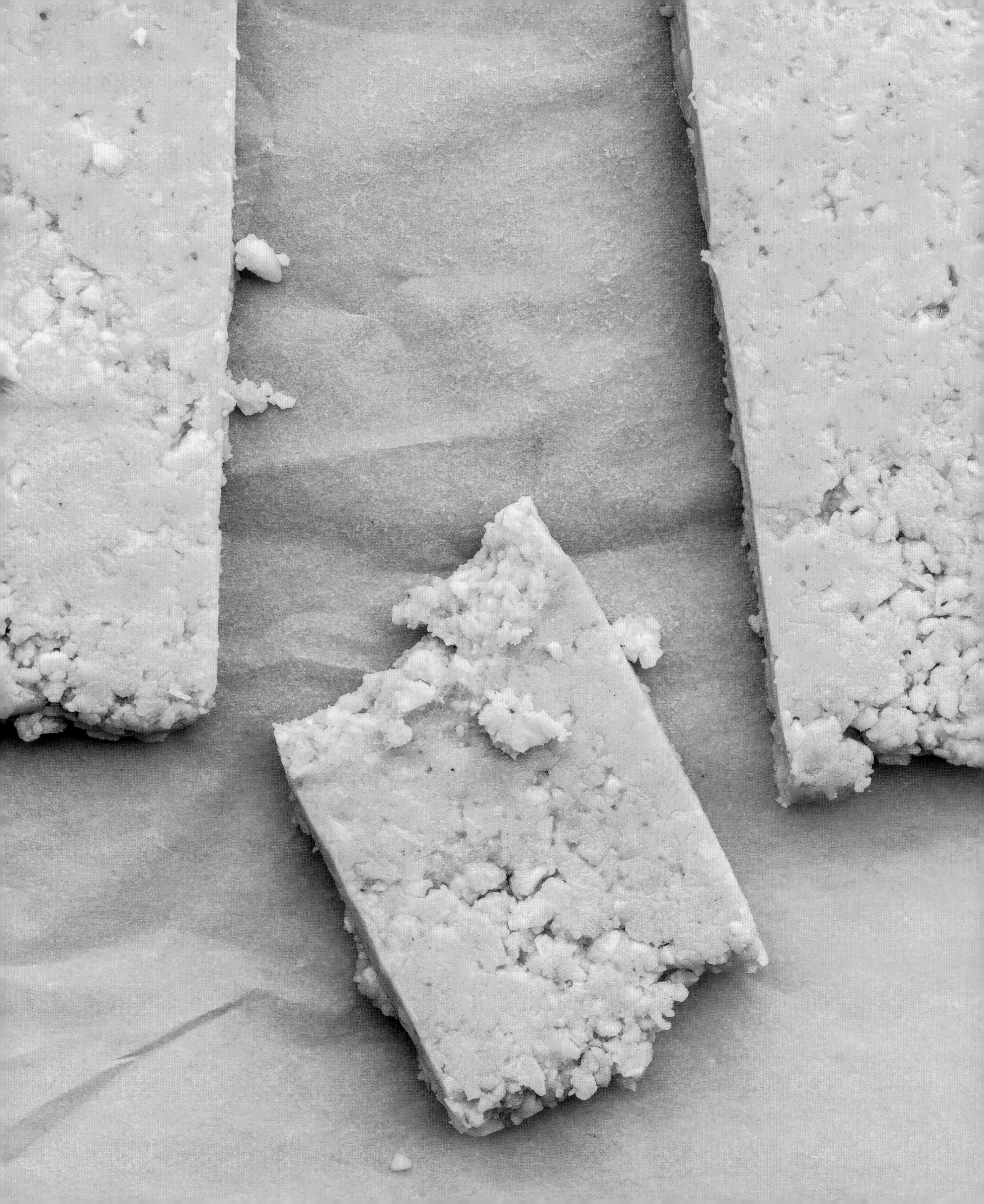

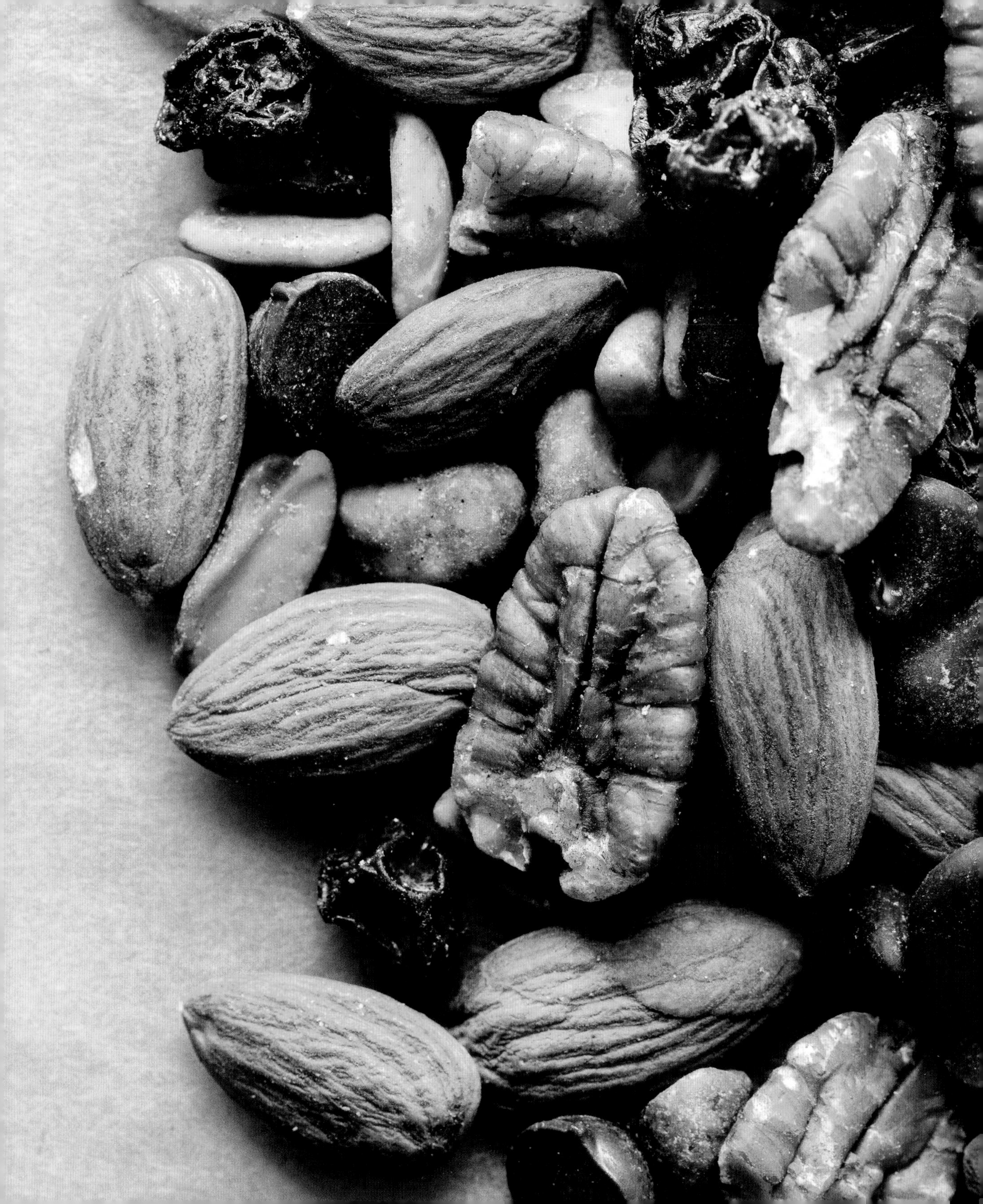

blood sugar–friendly nutty trail mix

What comes to mind when you think of trail mix? Most varieties include some sort of dried fruit and candy, which are not good for balancing blood sugars. But this recipe combines some of my favorite nuts and just a small amount of sweetness for a much more blood sugar–friendly option.

gluten-free | sodium aware | vegan | yield: 4 servings

¼ cup (31 g) raw shelled pistachios

¼ cup (30 g) raw pecans

¼ cup (43 g) raw almonds

¼ cup (38 g) raisins

¼ cup (45 g) dairy-free dark chocolate chips

In a medium bowl, combine the pistachios, pecans, almonds, raisins, and chocolate chips.

Divide the trail mix into four portions.

STORAGE: Store the trail mix in an airtight container in the pantry for up to 3 months.

Estimated Nutrition Facts per Serving: 234 calories; 21 g carbs; 4 g fiber; 15 g sugar; 5 g protein; 17 g fat (4 g saturated fat); 6 mg sodium

lemon cream fruit dip

This dip is the perfect sweet treat to enjoy with berries or whole-grain crackers. Most fruit dips are loaded with refined sugars and lacking in protein. But one serving of this Lemon Cream Fruit Dip gives you 7 grams of protein, thanks to the Greek yogurt, and it has only 80 calories! That protein makes it the perfect accompaniment for your favorite carbohydrate source, like crackers, pretzels, and fruit.

gluten-free | low carb | sodium aware | yield: 4 servings

1 cup (200 g) plain nonfat Greek yogurt

¼ cup (28 g) coconut flour

1 tbsp (15 ml) pure maple syrup

½ tsp pure vanilla extract

½ tsp pure almond extract

Zest of 1 medium lemon

Juice of ½ medium lemon

In a medium bowl, whisk together the yogurt, coconut flour, maple syrup, vanilla, almond extract, lemon zest, and lemon juice. Serve the dip with fruit or crackers.

STORAGE: Store the dip in a sealed container in the refrigerator for up to 1 week.

Estimated Nutrition Facts per Serving: 80 calories; 10 g carbs; 3 g fiber; 6 g sugar; 7 g protein; 1 g fat (1 g saturated fat); 37 mg sodium

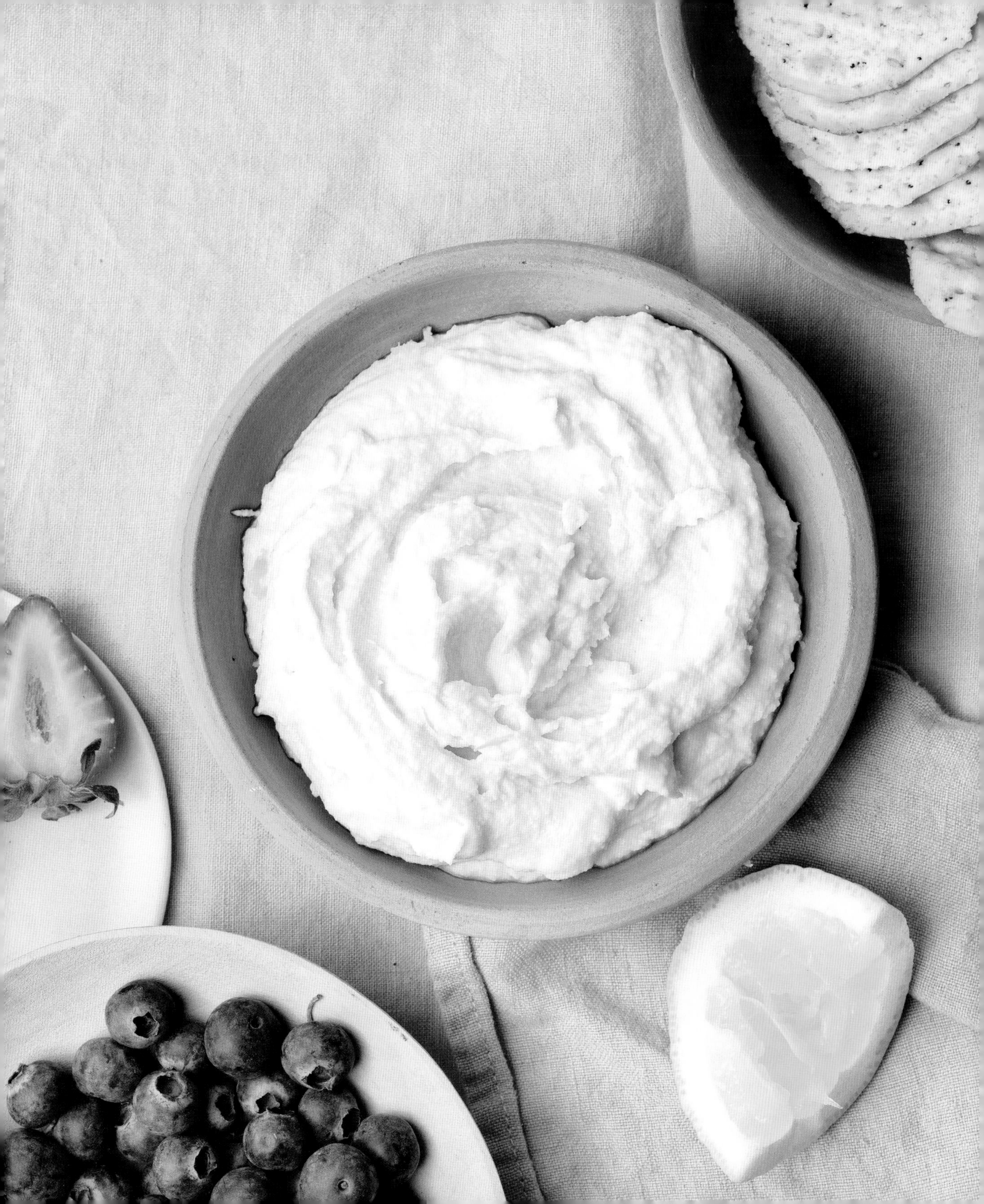

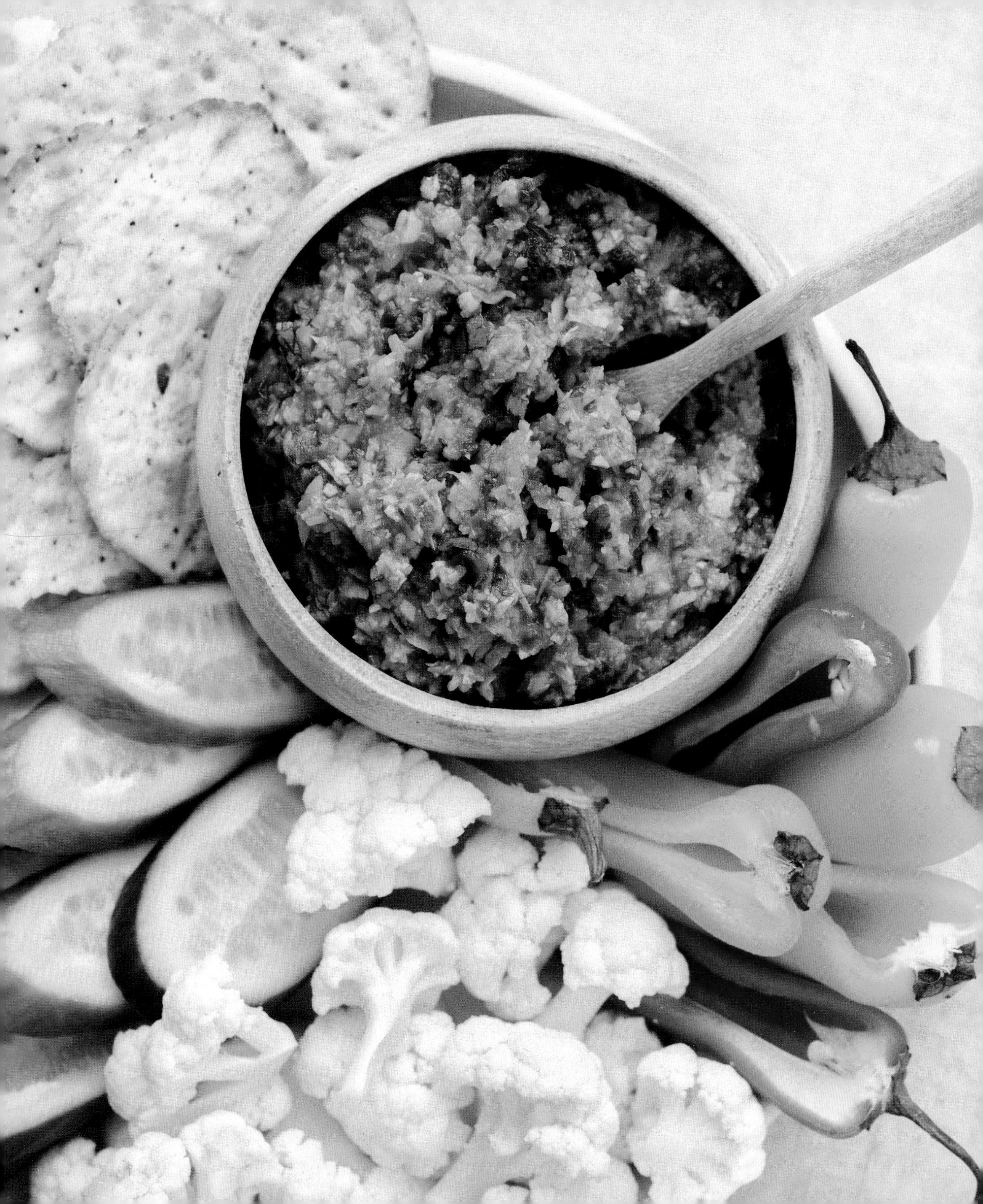

homemade sun-dried tomato salsa

Imagine your favorite antipasto platter blended into a delicious salsa! Artichokes are high in fiber and bring a unique twist to traditional salsa. So not only do we get amazing flavor with this recipe but we also get stable blood sugars. This salsa is delicious over cooked fish or chicken or as a dip with your favorite veggies. I love it with carrots, cucumbers, or raw cauliflower.

gluten-free | low carb | no added sugar | vegan | yield: 4 servings

½ (15-oz [425-g]) can no-salt-added diced tomatoes, drained

6 tbsp (20 g) julienned sun-dried tomatoes (see Tip)

1½ cups (330 g) canned artichoke hearts, drained

1 clove garlic

⅛ cup (3 g) fresh basil leaves

1 tsp balsamic vinegar

2 tbsp (30 ml) olive oil

Sea salt, as needed

Black pepper, as needed

In a food processor or blender, combine the diced tomatoes, sun-dried tomatoes, artichoke hearts, garlic, basil, vinegar, oil, sea salt, and black pepper. Process or blend the ingredients to the desired consistency.

STORAGE: Store the salsa in a sealed container in the refrigerator for up to 1 week.

TIP: This recipe calls for packaged julienned sun-dried tomatoes, not the jarred variety packed in oil. However, if you are unable to find packaged sun-dried tomatoes, you can substitute the oil-packed kind, but use just 1 tablespoon (15 ml) of olive oil.

Estimated Nutrition Facts per Serving: 131 calories; 13 g carbs; 4 g fiber; 3 g sugar; 2 g protein; 7 g fat (1 g saturated fat); 279 mg sodium

homemade movie night popcorn

Did you know popcorn has 4 grams of fiber per serving? Most people are surprised to learn it can be a very blood sugar–friendly snack if prepared properly. Go beyond buttered popcorn and skip the microwave stuff with these creative twists on the classic movie theater treat.

everything bagel popcorn: no added sugar | sodium aware | vegan
cinnamon-maple popcorn: sodium aware | vegan
savory popcorn: no added sugar | sodium aware
trail mix popcorn: sodium aware | vegan
yield: 4 servings

popcorn

1 tbsp (15 ml) avocado oil (see Tips)

½ cup (96 g) yellow popcorn kernels

everything bagel popcorn

2 tsp (6 g) everything bagel seasoning (see Tips)

cinnamon-maple popcorn

1 tsp ground cinnamon

2 tsp (10 ml) pure maple syrup

Sea salt, as needed

savory popcorn

2 tsp (2 g) dried rosemary

¼ cup (25 g) grated Parmesan cheese

Sea salt, as needed

Black pepper, as needed

trail mix popcorn

2 tbsp (22 g) dairy-free dark chocolate chips

2 tbsp (19 g) raisins

¼ cup (28 g) sliced almonds

To make the popcorn, heat the oil in a large lidded pot over medium-high heat for 2 to 3 minutes. Add three or four popcorn kernels to the pot and cover the pot with the lid. As soon as one of the kernels pops, add the remaining kernels.

Slightly tilt the lid to vent the steam and shake the pot occasionally, cooking the popcorn for about 3 minutes, until all the kernels have popped or the popping has slowed to every 1 to 2 seconds.

Remove the pot from the heat and add the ingredients of the desired flavor of popcorn, tossing to combine everything. Serve the popcorn hot.

STORAGE: Once the popcorn has cooled, store it in an airtight bag for up to 3 days.

TIPS: You may need to add a bit more oil to the cooked popcorn to help the seasonings stick.

You can buy premade everything bagel seasoning, or you can make your own by combining equal amounts of garlic powder, onion powder, poppy seeds, and sesame seeds with half the amount of flaky sea salt.

Estimated Nutrition Facts per Serving: Everything Bagel Popcorn: 126 calories; 17 g carbs; 4 g fiber; 0 g sugar; 3 g protein; 5 g fat; 118 mg sodium
Cinnamon-Maple Popcorn: 129 calories; 20 g carbs; 4 g fiber; 2 g sugar; 3 g protein; 5 g fat; 0 mg sodium
Savory Popcorn: 147 calories; 17 g carbs; 4 g fiber; 0 g sugar; 5 g protein; 7 g fat (2 g saturated fat); 46 mg sodium
Trail Mix Popcorn: 218 calories; 26 g carbs; 4 g fiber; 7 g sugar; 5 g protein; 11 g fat (3 g saturated fat); 4 mg sodium

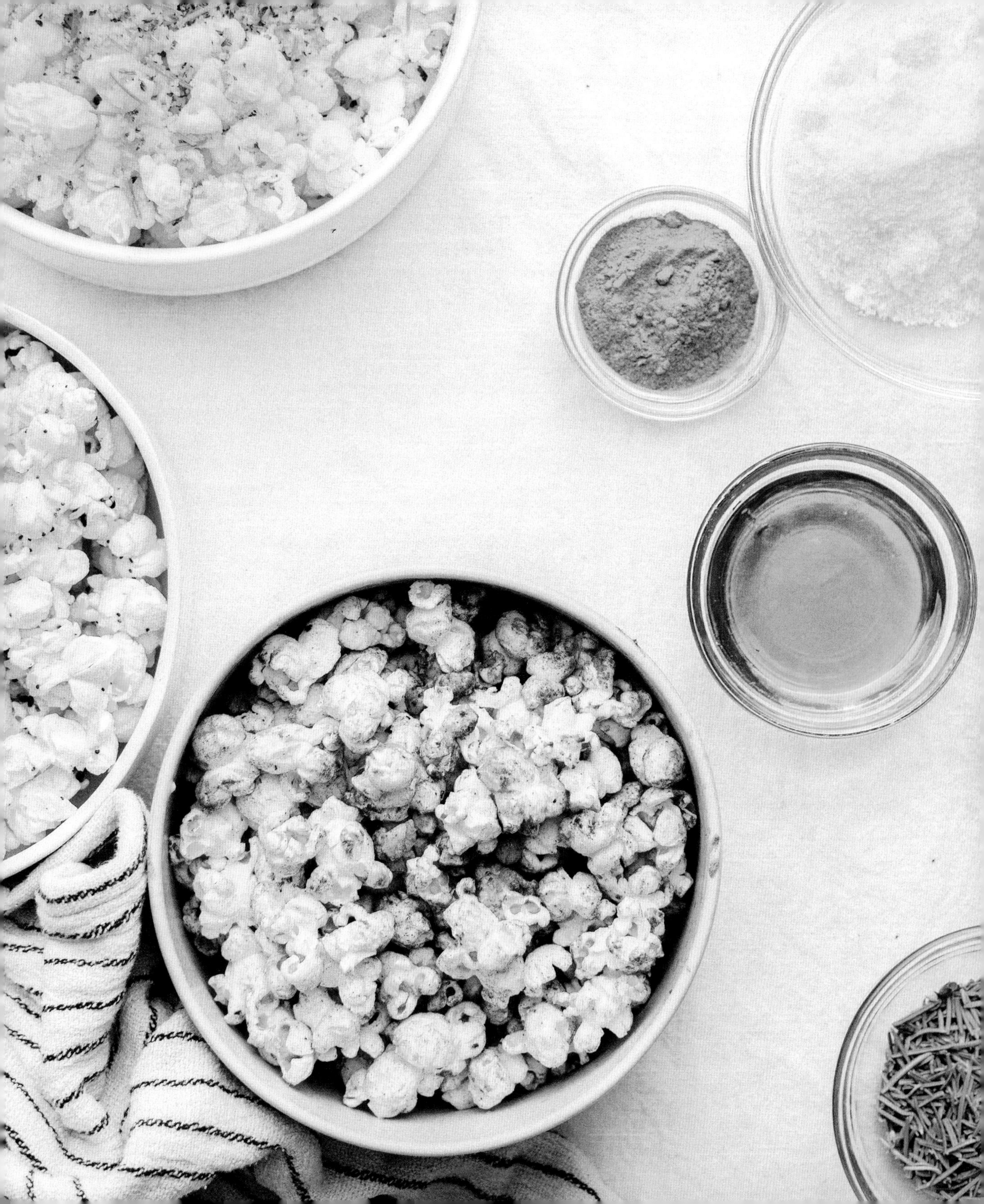

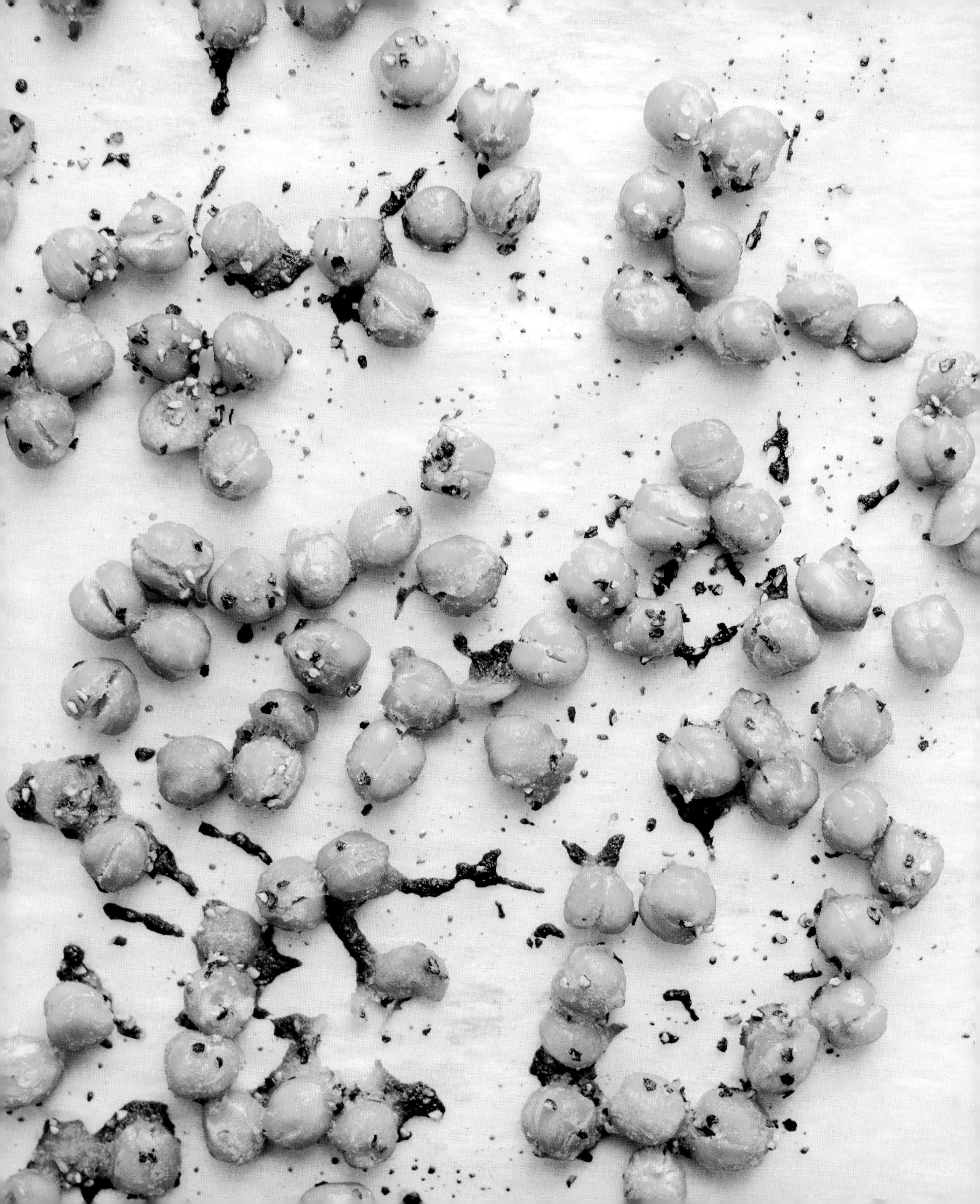

tangy roasted chickpeas

Give your favorite crunchy snack a fiber and protein upgrade in this quick and easy recipe. Chickpeas morph into a satisfying crunchy snack in the oven and taste great by the handful. Their natural fiber and protein content means they're a crunchy snack that will also keep blood sugars steady between meals.

gluten-free | sodium aware | yield: 4 servings

1 (15-oz [425-g]) can chickpeas, drained and rinsed

2 tsp (6 g) yellow mustard

1 tsp garlic powder

Sea salt, as needed

Black pepper, as needed

1 tbsp (15 ml) olive oil

1 tsp honey or agave nectar

1 tbsp (15 ml) water

Preheat the oven to 400°F (204°C). Line a large baking sheet with parchment paper.

Place the chickpeas between two kitchen towels and rub them until they are dry and most of the translucent skins have been removed. This step will make them extra crispy.

In a large bowl, whisk together the mustard, garlic powder, sea salt, black pepper, oil, honey, and water. Add the chickpeas, stirring to evenly coat them. Spread the chickpeas out evenly on the prepared baking sheet.

Bake the chickpeas for 25 minutes, until they are golden brown and crispy. Let them cool for 10 to 15 minutes before serving.

STORAGE: Store the chickpeas in an airtight container in the refrigerator for up to 1 week.

Estimated Nutrition Facts per Serving: 128 calories; 17 g carbs; 4 g fiber; 4 g sugar; 5 g protein; 5 g fat (1 g saturated fat); 46 mg sodium

no-added-sugar berries and cream yogurt bowl

Flavored yogurt cups often come loaded with added sugar and don't offer a significant source of protein. By making our own version at home, we've not only cut back on sugar but added 27 grams of protein. Less sugar and more protein means happy blood sugars!

gluten-free | no added sugar | protein packed | sodium aware | yield: 1 serving

1 cup (200 g) plain nonfat Greek yogurt

1 tbsp (15 g) almond butter

½ cup (50 g) frozen mixed berries, thawed

Zest of ½ medium lemon

In a small bowl, combine the yogurt, almond butter, berries, and lemon zest.

STORAGE: Eat this yogurt bowl immediately, or store it in a sealed container in the refrigerator for up to 2 days.

Estimated Nutrition Facts per Serving: 270 calories; 21 g carbs; 3 g fiber; 15 g sugar; 27 g protein; 10 g fat (1 g saturated fat); 89 mg sodium

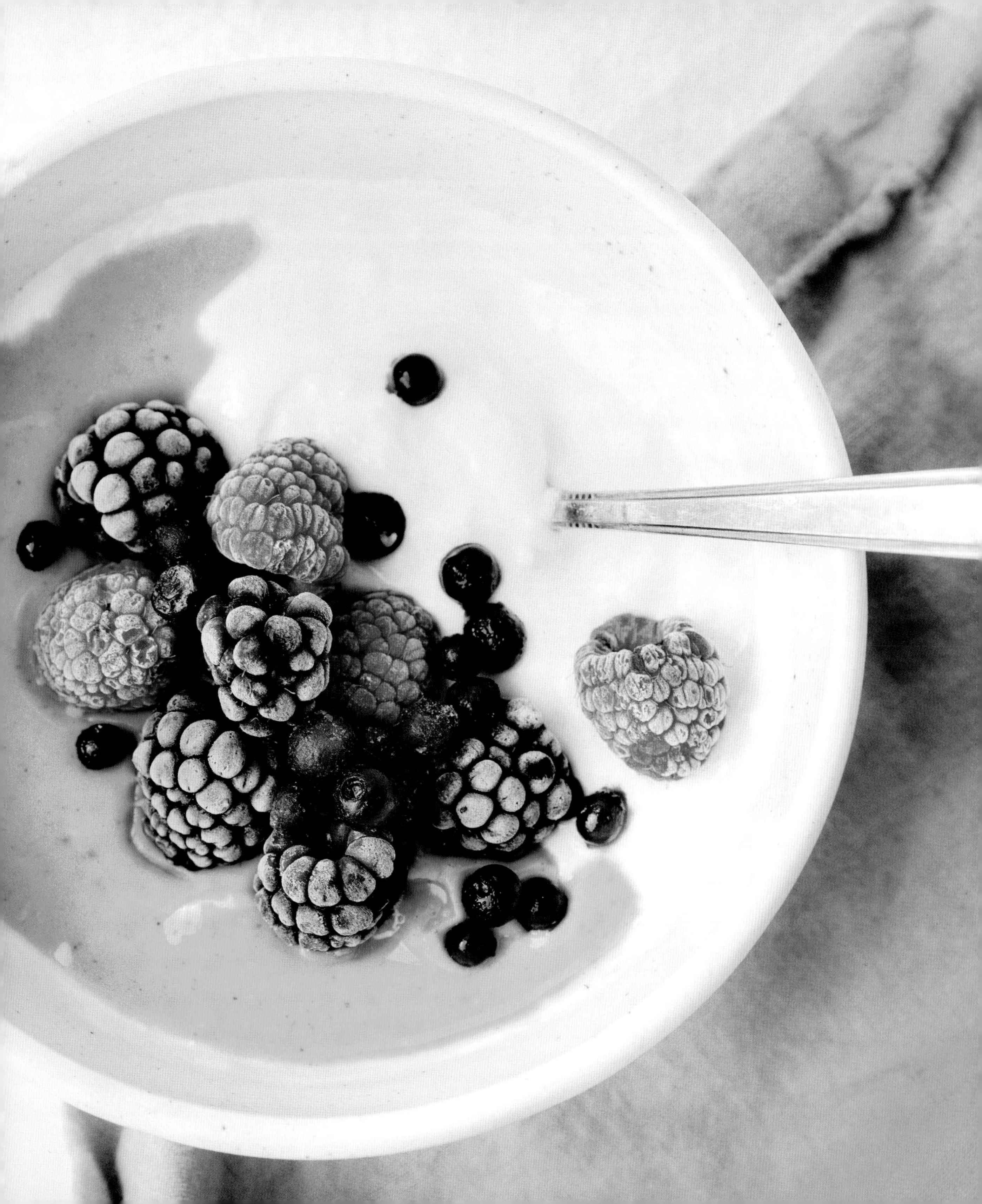

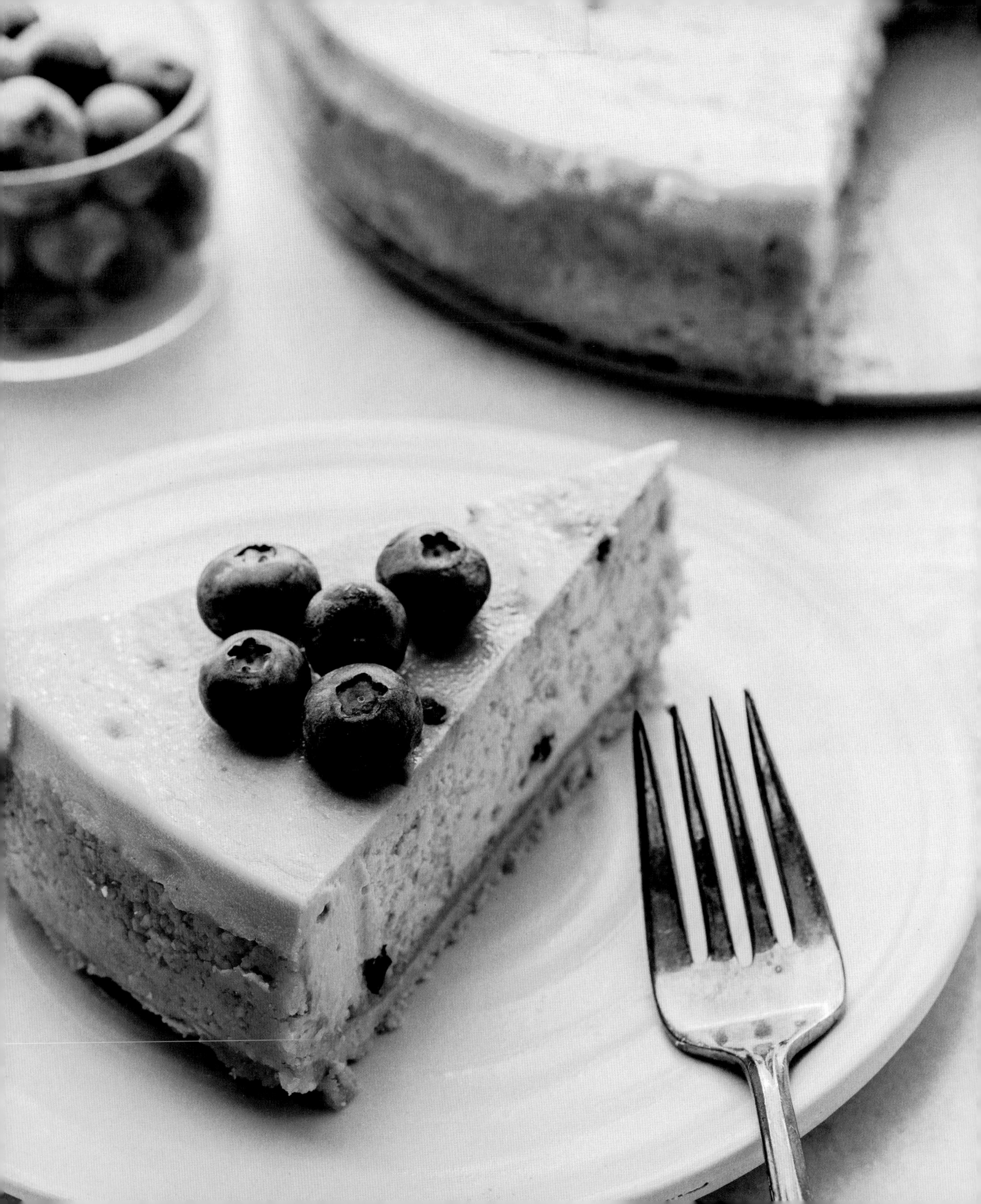

blood sugar–friendly desserts

LOW-SUGAR TREATS THAT WILL SATISFY ANYONE'S SWEET TOOTH

Believe it or not, it is possible to make delicious low-sugar desserts that are blood sugar–friendly and taste like the "real thing." The recipes in this chapter are perfect for celebrations or just because and will satisfy that sweet tooth we all have from time to time.

There are a few things I try to do when creating recipes for blood sugar–friendly desserts:

- I use grain-free flours or ground nuts instead of traditional grain-based flours. Grain-free flours have fewer carbohydrates and more protein and fat than traditional flours.
- I focus on low-sugar mix-ins or toppings. These include things like nuts, seeds, fresh fruit, or nut butters.
- I use less sugar, syrup, or sweetener. Most recipes don't actually need as much sugar as they call for to taste sweet. For example, you can usually cut the sugar by half in a typical cookie recipe and still have just as tasty a cookie.
- I look for (or create) recipes I think I'm actually going to like. It's important to focus on flavors you love. Don't force yourself to eat something that you think you won't enjoy or that you aren't looking forward to.

Whether you try the Flourless Chocolate Chip–Pecan Cookies (page 129) or the Strawberry Cheesecake in a Jar (page 133), these dessert recipes will help you satisfy your sweet tooth without spiking your blood sugars.

flourless chocolate chip–pecan cookies

When was the last time you had a chocolate chip cookie that had only 6 grams of sugar? Well, these cookies are not only blood sugar–friendly, but the rich pecan flavor will leave your taste buds singing! And don't be afraid to make mini cookies—just cut down on the baking time by three or four minutes.

gluten-free | low carb | sodium aware | yield: 18 cookies

2 cups (218 g) coarsely chopped pecans or pecan pieces

1 cup (80 g) gluten-free rolled oats

⅓ cup (77 g) unsalted butter or coconut oil

⅓ cup (80 ml) pure maple syrup

1 tsp ground cinnamon

¼ tsp sea salt

½ tsp baking soda

2 tsp (10 ml) pure vanilla extract

1 tsp pure almond extract

½ cup (90 g) dark chocolate chips

Preheat the oven to 350°F (177°C). Line a large baking sheet with parchment paper.

In a food processor, combine the pecans and oats. Process them until a powder forms. Add the butter and pulse until the ingredients are well combined. Add the maple syrup, cinnamon, sea salt, baking soda, vanilla, and almond extract. Process the ingredients for 20 to 30 seconds, until a dough forms. Be careful not to overprocess the dough, as processing the dough for too long can make it too wet because the oils separate from the pecans.

Carefully remove the blade from the food processor and stir in the chocolate chips by hand.

Using a cookie scoop or a 1-tablespoon (15-g) measure, scoop the dough into balls and place them on the prepared baking sheet. Bake the cookies for 12 to 14 minutes, or until they are set and the tops are golden.

Remove the cookies from the oven and let them cool for 4 to 5 minutes before transferring them to a wire rack to finish cooling.

STORAGE: Store the cookies in an airtight container for up to 1 week, or freeze them for up to 3 months.

Estimated Nutrition Facts per Serving (1 cookie): 190 calories; 12 g carbs; 2 g fiber; 6 g sugar; 2 g protein; 16 g fat (6 g saturated fat); 69 mg sodium

peanut butter fudge brownies

A dense, fudgy brownie is one of my favorite sweet treats. This version has only 11 grams of sugar and 3 grams of protein per brownie. By using a combination of almond flour and oats, we create the perfect brownie texture that's also lower in carbohydrates and higher in fiber than traditional flour. Make this recipe and you'll learn to love brownies again!

gluten-free | sodium aware | vegan | yield: 12 brownies

Cooking oil spray, as needed

1 cup (80 g) gluten-free rolled oats

½ cup (48 g) almond flour

1 cup (194 g) canned low-sodium black beans, drained and rinsed

¼ cup (60 ml) cooking oil of choice

1½ tsp (8 ml) pure vanilla extract

¼ tsp baking soda

1 tsp baking powder

¼ tsp sea salt

1 tsp ground cinnamon

⅓ cup (32 g) unsweetened cocoa powder

½ cup (120 ml) pure maple syrup

¼ cup (45 g) dairy-free dark chocolate chips

2 tbsp (30 g) all-natural peanut butter (see Tip)

Preheat the oven to 350°F (177°C). Spray an 8 x 8–inch (20 x 20–cm) baking pan with the cooking oil spray.

In a food processor, combine the oats, almond flour, beans, oil, vanilla, baking soda, baking powder, sea salt, cinnamon, cocoa powder, and maple syrup. Process the ingredients for about 1 minute, until the batter is smooth. You may need to stop the food processor once and scrape down the sides.

Carefully remove the food processor's blade and stir in the chocolate chips by hand.

Spread the batter into the prepared baking pan. Drizzle the peanut butter over the top of the batter.

Bake the brownies for 15 minutes, until a toothpick inserted into the center comes out clean. Let the brownies cool completely in the pan on a wire rack.

STORAGE: Store the brownies in an airtight container for up to 3 days, or freeze them for up to 3 months.

TIP: Be sure to buy an all-natural peanut butter with no added salt or sugar.

Estimated Nutrition Facts per Serving (1 brownie): 170 calories; 19 g carbs; 2 g fiber; 11 g sugar; 3 g protein; 10 g fat (2 g saturated fat); 52 mg sodium

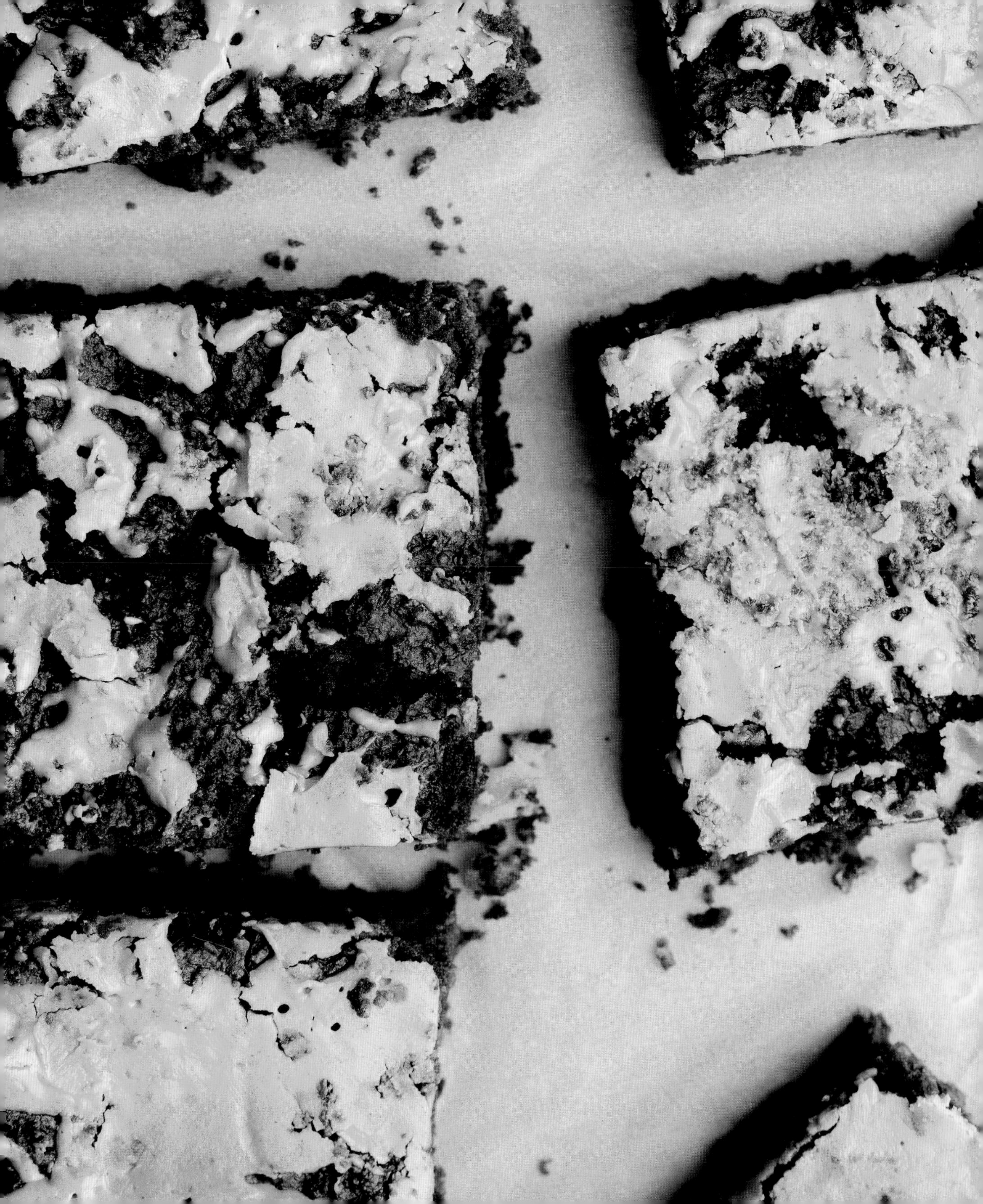

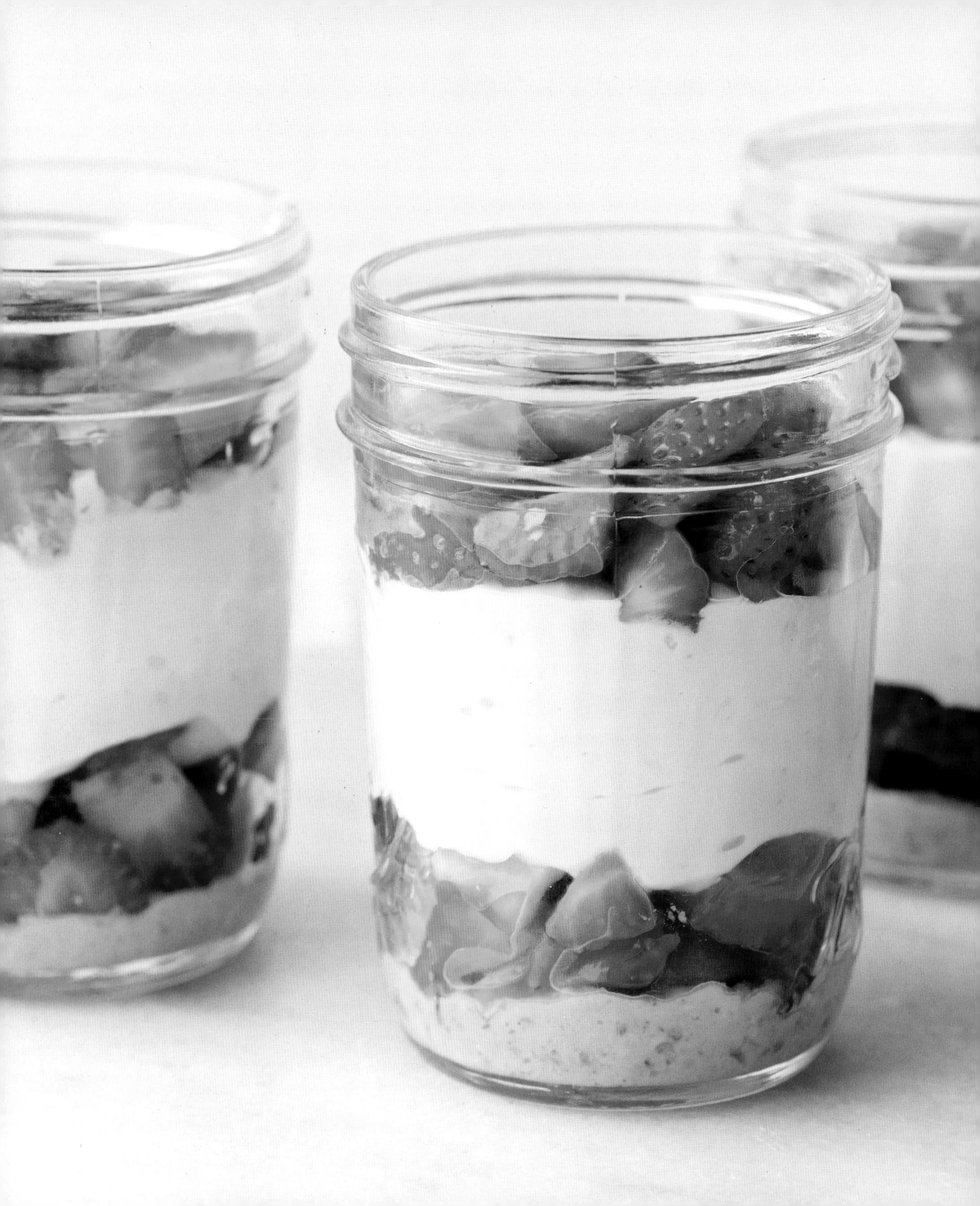

strawberry cheesecake in a jar

This no-bake dessert is perfect any time of year, but it makes the perfect summertime treat. The rich, buttery crust has no added sugar and is packed with plant-based fats that help stabilize blood sugars much better than traditional pie or cheesecake crusts. The filling is made with a lightened-up combination of cream cheese, plain Greek yogurt, and other flavorings that are loaded with deliciousness—but not sugar!

gluten-free | sodium aware | yield: 8 servings

½ cup (55 g) raw cashews

¼ cup (60 g) all-natural peanut butter

2 tbsp (12 g) almond flour

1 large pitted Medjool date

1 cup (200 g) coarsely chopped strawberries, plus more as needed

8 oz (227 g) cream cheese

½ cup (100 g) plain nonfat Greek yogurt

¼ cup (60 ml) pure maple syrup

Zest of 1 medium lemon, plus more as needed

1 tbsp (15 ml) pure vanilla extract

In a food processor, combine the cashews, peanut butter, almond flour, and Medjool date. Process the ingredients until a dough forms.

Divide the dough among eight (8-oz [227-ml]) mason jars. Press the dough down into each jar to make a crust.

Divide the strawberries among the jars on top of the crusts.

In a food processor or high-power blender, combine the cream cheese, yogurt, maple syrup, lemon zest, and vanilla. Process the ingredients until they are smooth.

Divide the cheesecake mixture evenly among the jars, tapping them gently on the counter to shake out all the air bubbles.

Top the cheesecakes with additional strawberries and lemon zest if desired.

Refrigerate the cheesecakes for at least 2 hours or overnight before serving.

STORAGE: Store the cheesecakes, covered, in the refrigerator for up to 5 days.

Estimated Nutrition Facts per Serving: 253 calories; 17 g carbs; 2 g fiber; 12 g sugar; 7 g protein; 18 g fat (8 g saturated fat); 115 mg sodium

crispy pistachio chocolate bark

Dark chocolate is not only an antioxidant powerhouse but it also typically has less sugar and more flavor than other varieties of chocolate. This chocolate bark recipe is a lower-sugar version of your favorite chocolate treat!

gluten-free | low carb | sodium aware | vegan | yield: 16 servings

1 cup (180 g) dairy-free 70% dark chocolate chips, melted

¼ cup (6 g) crisped rice cereal

½ cup (50 g) crushed pistachios

Line a large baking sheet with parchment paper.

In a medium bowl, combine the chocolate and rice cereal and stir to combine.

Spread the mixture out evenly on the prepared baking sheet to your desired thickness. I recommend ¼ inch (6 mm).

Sprinkle the pistachios on top of the chocolate mixture and press them lightly with your hands or the back of a spoon to ensure that they stick to the chocolate.

Place the bark in the freezer for 1 hour.

Remove the bark from the freezer and break it into 16 pieces.

STORAGE: Store the bark in an airtight container in the refrigerator for up to 1 month.

Estimated Nutrition Facts per Serving: 101 calories; 11 g carbs; 2 g fiber; 8 g sugar; 2 g protein; 7 g fat (3 g saturated fat); 8 mg sodium

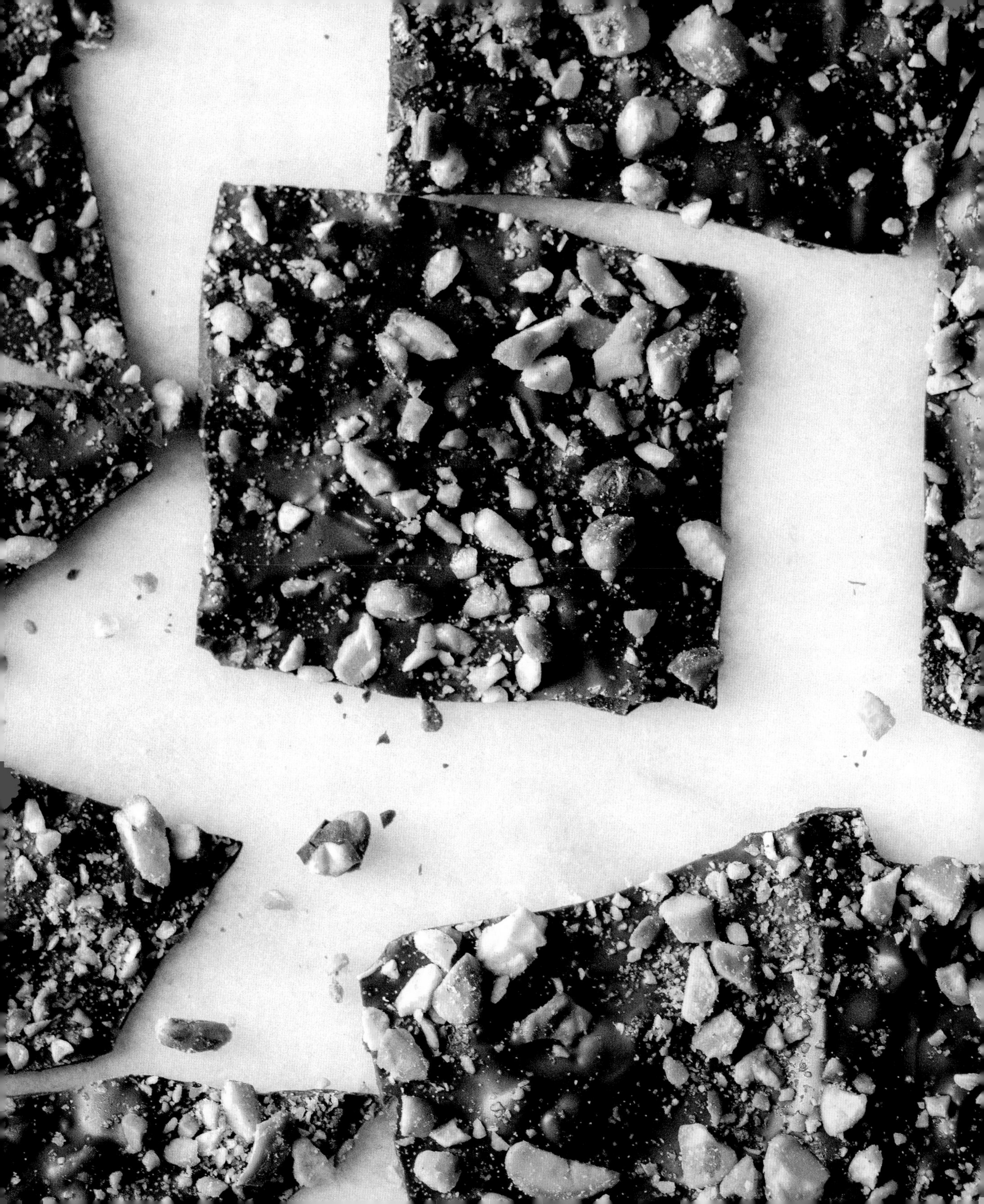

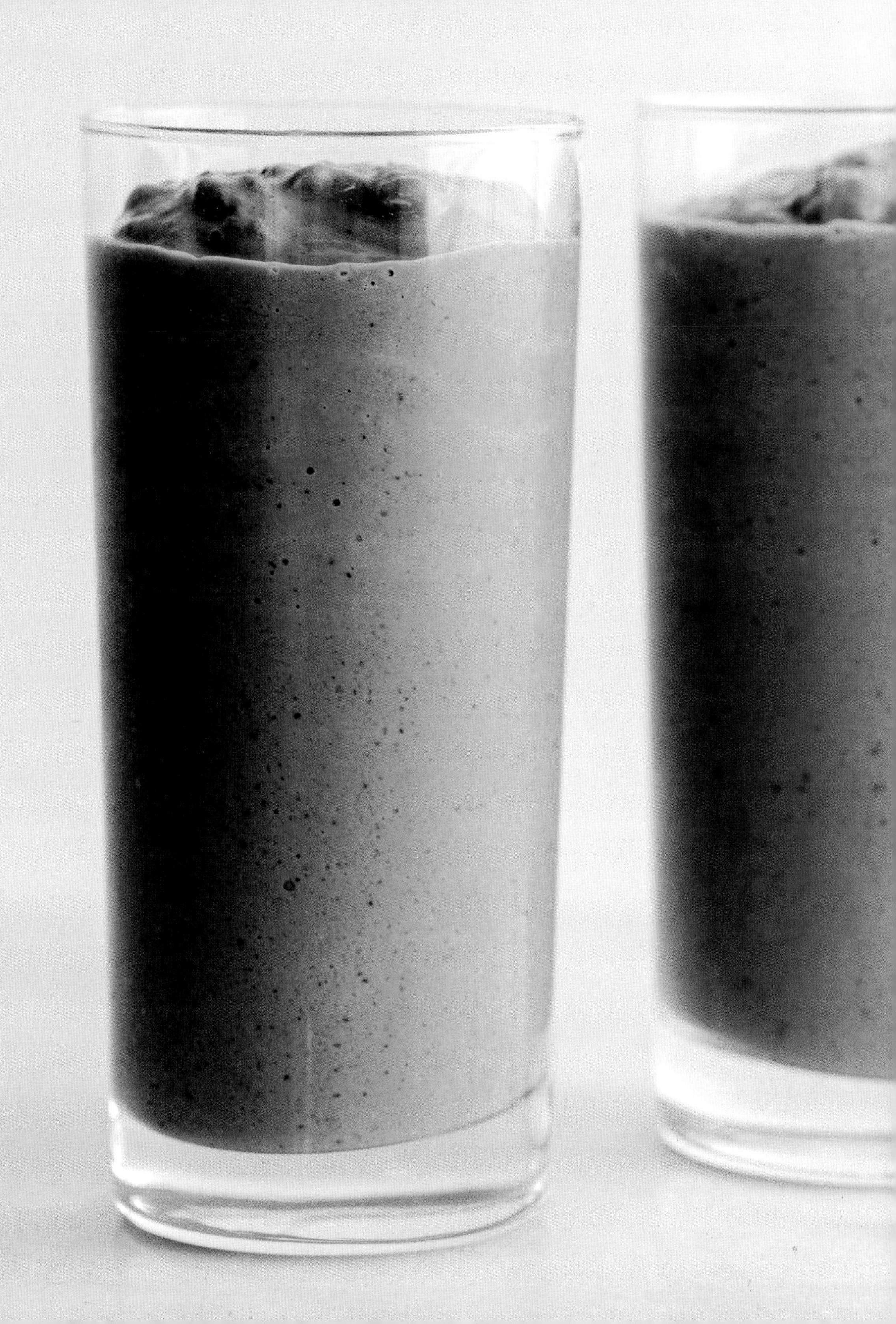

frozen mocha milkshake

This Frozen Mocha Milkshake will make you think you're at your favorite coffee shop or ice cream parlor. The surprise ingredient, avocado, not only adds creaminess but a hefty dose of fiber too! With both plant-based fat and fiber, it's got a leg up on that coffeehouse version and won't leave your blood sugars skyrocketing like a traditional milkshake would.

gluten-free | high fiber | sodium aware | vegan | yield: 1 serving

1 cup (240 ml) unsweetened vanilla almond milk

3 tbsp (18 g) unsweetened cocoa powder

2 tsp (4 g) instant espresso powder

1½ cups (210 g) crushed ice

½ medium avocado, peeled and pitted

1 tbsp (15 ml) pure maple syrup

1 tsp pure vanilla extract

In a blender, combine the almond milk, cocoa powder, espresso powder, ice, avocado, maple syrup, and vanilla. Blend the ingredients on high speed for 60 seconds, until the milkshake is smooth.

STORAGE: Enjoy this milkshake immediately.

Estimated Nutrition Facts per Serving: 307 calories; 33 g carbs; 13 g fiber; 13 g sugar; 6 g protein; 20 g fat (4 g saturated fat); 173 mg sodium

low-sugar blueberry swirl cheesecake

Cheesecake started it all for me. It was the first thing my grandmother taught me how to make and the first thing I learned how to make with less sugar that still tasted delicious! This recipe is a variation on the classic low-sugar cheesecake recipe I've been making since I was 12 years old in my grandma's kitchen.

gluten-free | sodium aware | yield: 16 servings

2 cups (220 g) raw cashews

½ cup (120 g) nut butter of choice

3 (8-oz [227-g]) packages light cream cheese, at room temperature

¾ cup (144 g) coconut sugar

3 large eggs, at room temperature

1½ cups (300 g) plain nonfat Greek yogurt, at room temperature

2 tsp (10 ml) pure vanilla extract, at room temperature

1 cup (150 g) frozen blueberries, thawed (see Tips)

Water, as needed

Preheat the oven to 325°F (163°C). Wrap a springform pan in several layers of foil.

In a food processor, combine the cashews and nut butter. Process the ingredients until a dough forms. Press the dough into the prepared springform pan, either on the bottom only or up the sides as well as the bottom. Set the pan aside.

Using a stand mixer or hand mixer fitted with a whisk attachment, beat the cream cheese and coconut sugar for about 1 minute, until the mixture is fluffy. Add the eggs one at a time and beat the mixture after each addition to incorporate the egg. Add the yogurt and vanilla and beat the mixture one last time to incorporate the ingredients. Mix half of the blueberries into the batter by hand. Pour the cheesecake batter into the crust.

Add the remaining blueberries on top of the batter and lightly swirl them around the top, gently mixing them into the batter.

Place the springform pan inside of a larger pan. Add the water to the larger pan until it is about halfway up the side of the springform pan. This water bath will help ensure the sides of the cheesecake maintain a constant temperature while baking.

Bake the cheesecake for 90 minutes, or until it is set but still jiggles slightly. Remove the cheesecake from the oven and out of the water bath. Let the cheesecake cool to room temperature. Once it has cooled, place the cheesecake in the refrigerator for at least 4 hours before eating.

STORAGE: This cheesecake will keep in the refrigerator for up to 1 week and in the freezer for up to 1 month.

Estimated Nutrition Facts per Serving: 304 calories; 18 g carbs; 1 g fiber; 13 g sugar; 10 g protein; 21 g fat (9 g saturated fat); 207 mg sodium

TIPS: I like to use frozen blueberries that have thawed because of the yummy juice that leaks out of the berries. It adds to the texture and visual appeal of the cheesecake!

To prevent the top of the cheesecake from cracking, have all of your ingredients at room temperature before starting.

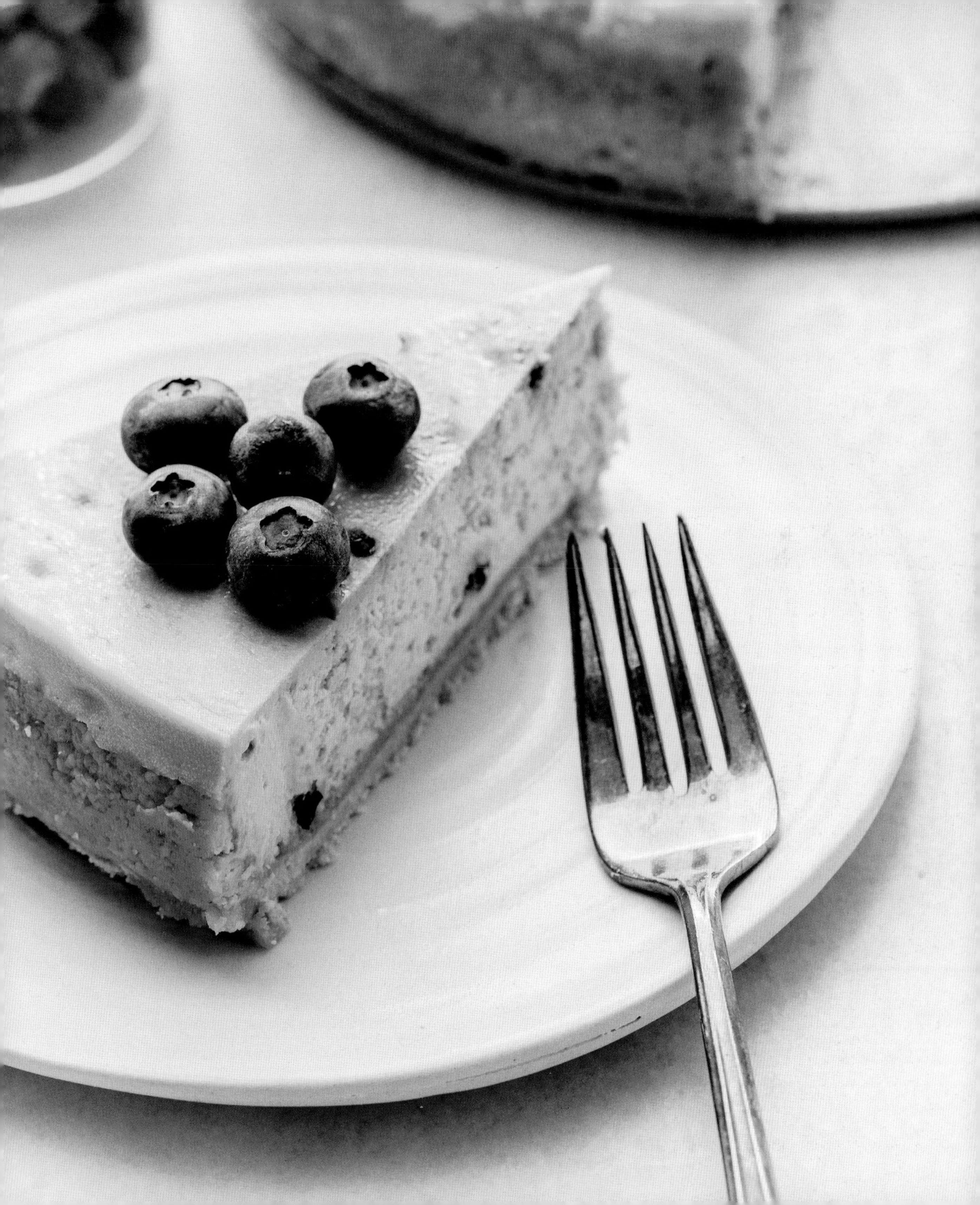

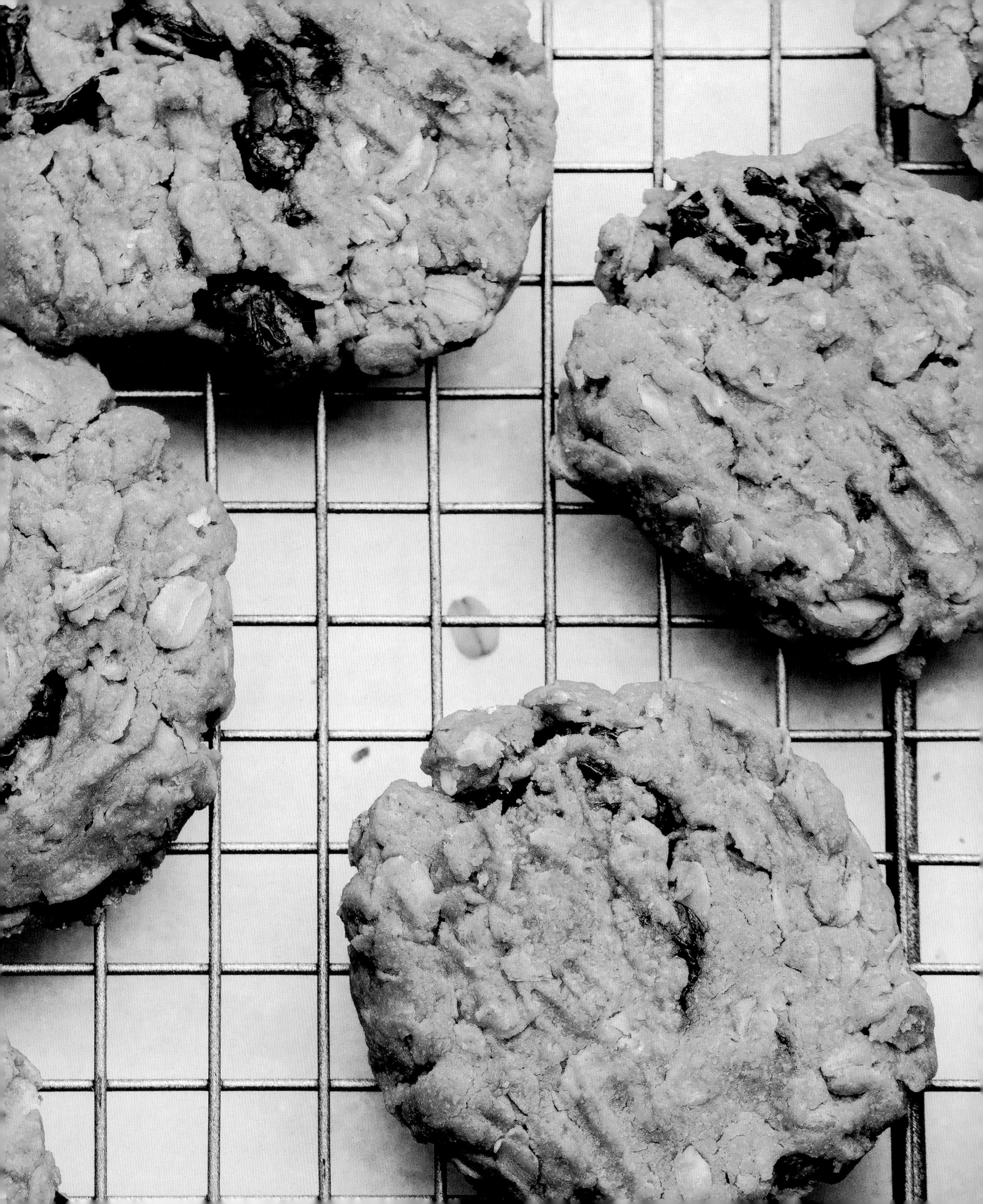

5-ingredient chunky cherry and peanut butter cookies

A cookie that also packs 7 grams of protein? Yes, please! These simple cookies not only taste great but with their fat, fiber, and protein content, they are a great blood sugar–friendly sweet treat for any time of day. They're less sweet than a traditional cookie, so they also make a wonderful breakfast cookie.

gluten-free | sodium aware | yield: 12 cookies

1 cup (240 g) all-natural peanut butter

¼ cup (60 ml) pure maple syrup

1 large egg, beaten

1 cup (80 g) gluten-free rolled or quick oats

½ cup (80 g) dried cherries

Preheat the oven to 350°F (177°C). Line a large baking sheet with parchment paper.

In a large bowl, whisk together the peanut butter, maple syrup, and egg. Add the oats and cherries, and mix until the ingredients are combined.

Chill the dough for 10 to 15 minutes.

Use a cookie scoop to scoop balls of the dough onto the prepared baking sheet.

Using a fork, gently flatten the dough balls into your desired shape (the cookies will not change shape much during baking). Bake the cookies for 10 to 12 minutes, until they are lightly golden on top.

Remove the cookies from the oven and let them cool for 5 minutes before transferring them to a wire rack.

STORAGE: Store the cookies in an airtight container for up to 3 days, or freeze them for up to 3 months.

Estimated Nutrition Facts per Serving: 198 calories; 19 g carbs; 3 g fiber; 11 g sugar; 7 g protein; 12 g fat (2 g saturated fat); 13 mg sodium

no-added-sugar orange and cream slushy

This recipe makes me think of summer, popsicles, lounging by the pool, and running through the sprinklers as a kid. There are certain foods and recipes that bring out a sense of nostalgia in all of us, and this is definitely one of those recipes for me. To put a better-for-your-blood-sugar spin on this classic treat, I've added some chia seeds and coconut for extra fiber and healthy fat!

gluten-free | high fiber | sodium aware | yield: 2 servings

½ cup (120 ml) unsweetened vanilla almond milk

½ cup (100 g) plain whole-milk yogurt

2 small oranges, peeled, seeds and pith removed, and frozen

1 small banana, frozen

1 tsp pure vanilla extract

2 tbsp (10 g) unsweetened coconut flakes

1 tbsp (12 g) chia seeds

In a high-power blender, combine the almond milk, yogurt, oranges, banana, vanilla, coconut flakes, and chia seeds. Blend the ingredients for 30 to 45 seconds, until a slushy consistency is reached.

STORAGE: Enjoy this slushy immediately.

Estimated Nutrition Facts per Serving: 203 calories; 29 g carbs; 7 g fiber; 17 g sugar; 8 g protein; 7 g fat (3 g saturated fat); 67 mg sodium

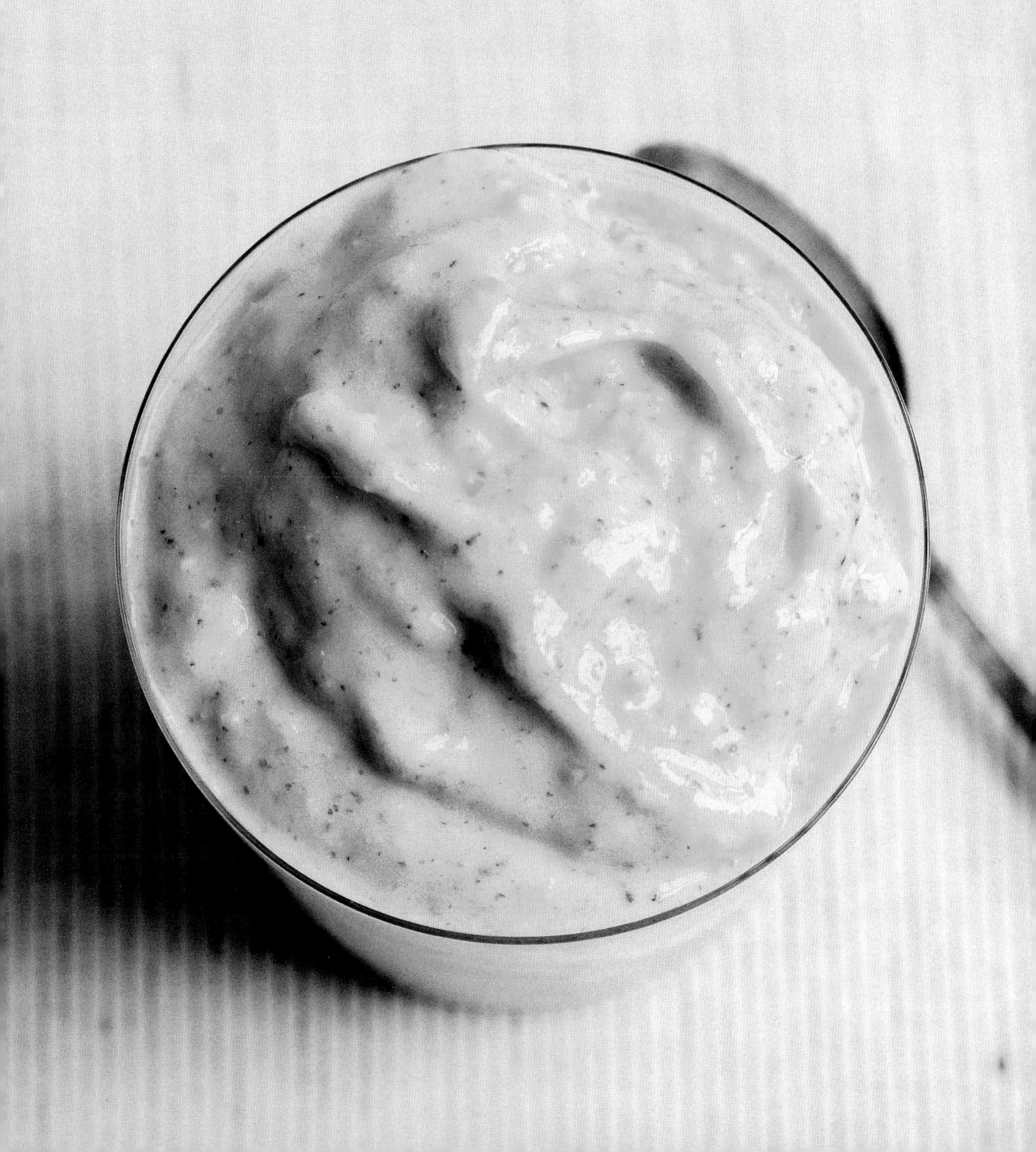

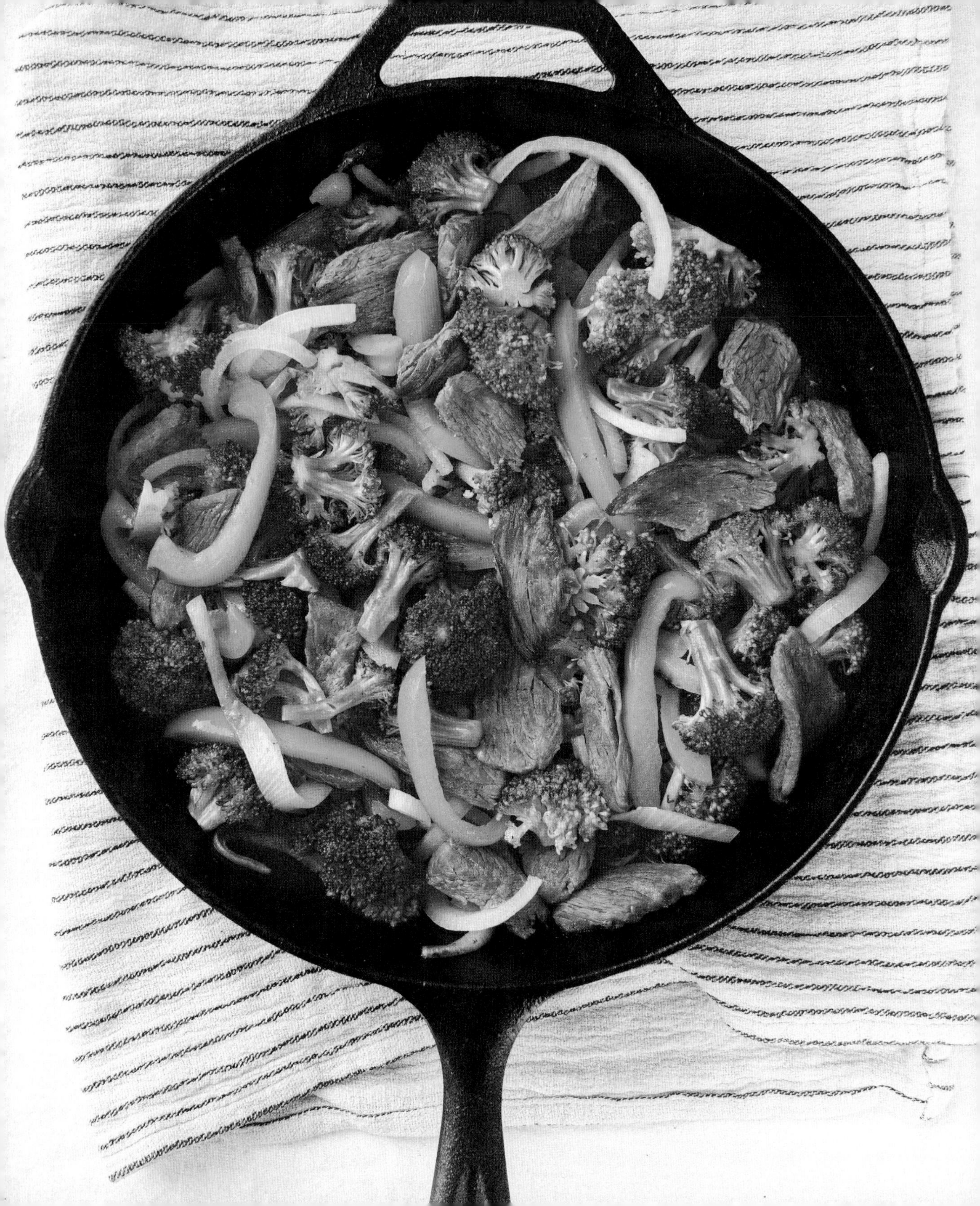

kitchen resources

STOCKING A DIABETES-FRIENDLY KITCHEN: EVERYTHING YOU NEED TO BE PREPARED

Whether you're cooking for yourself or a family member, there are certain foods and tools that make cooking for diabetes much easier. It's important to stock your kitchen, pantry, refrigerator, and freezer with all of the best, most nourishing ingredients and the most helpful, efficient tools. Now, I won't waste your time with general food items that everyone should have on hand, like fruits, veggies, and whole grains. The items in the following lists are specific to diabetes. These foods and tools make preparing and enjoying blood sugar–friendly foods both easier and tastier!

Pantry Staples

- **Grain-free flours:** Grain-free flours include things like almond flour and coconut flour. You likely noticed that I used both of these in most of the dessert recipes. Grain-free flours have a lower glycemic index than traditional white flour and even whole-wheat flour. They are higher in protein and fat and lower in total carbohydrates, which means they are ideal for blood sugar–friendly baked goods and other recipes. I advise anyone looking to manage blood sugars to always have these flours on hand and seek out recipes that use these flours over grain-based flours whenever possible.
- **Nuts, nut butters, seeds, and seed butters:** This category includes everything from pecans to chia seeds, cashews to peanut butter, and walnuts to pumpkin seeds. Both nuts and seeds are nutritional powerhouses that have a low glycemic index. They have all three of my favorite nutrients: fat, fiber, and protein. Adding them to dishes like baked goods, pastas, salads, and breakfast items can lower the glycemic impact of the overall meal, meaning they make it more blood sugar–friendly. I recommend raw or roasted nuts that do not have any salt or sugar added to them.
- **Popcorn:** Everyone loves a salty, crunchy snack at one point or another. Or maybe you want something to serve on the side of a sandwich or a casual meal. Potato chips can spike blood sugars quite easily, but popcorn has a higher fiber content and tends to keep you fuller longer. Keeping popcorn (that doesn't have a lot of salt or butter added) in your pantry allows you to still enjoy that salty snack you crave but also makes managing your blood sugars easier. Or keep popcorn kernels in your pantry and make your own, like my recipe on page 120 for Homemade Movie Night Popcorn.

- **Bean-based pastas:** Ever since bean-based pastas started to gain in popularity several years ago, I've always recommended them to people trying to balance blood sugars. Often pasta is the first thing most people with diabetes assume they have to give up, and many people are also the most upset about having to give up pasta. But with pastas made with everything from black beans to lentils to chickpeas now taking up a good chunk of the pasta aisle at every grocery store, I'm here to say you can still enjoy your favorite pasta dishes—like my Mediterranean Pasta Salad with Goat Cheese (page 72) or my Meatless Monday Spinach Lasagna (page 44)—while managing your blood sugars. Bean-based pastas have a higher protein content and lower carbohydrate content than traditional pasta.
- **Quinoa:** Quinoa is a great, tasty alternative to rice for people with diabetes. Rice—yes, even brown rice—can be very tricky for people with diabetes to enjoy. Because of the lack of fat, fiber, and protein, even the smallest amount can wreak havoc on blood sugars. But quinoa is much friendlier to blood sugars and has a similar cooking time to rice. It also has a lower carbohydrate content and a higher protein content than rice. Whether you replace all of the rice in a recipe with quinoa or just half, it is definitely a food I recommend keeping on hand.
- **Vanilla extract and almond extract:** Both of these extracts can lend a sweeter flavor and a more enjoyable eating experience to dishes without adding additional sugar and carbohydrates to dishes. You can often "sweeten up" everything from baked goods to yogurt bowls to smoothies with extracts and not have to rely on alternative sweeteners or additional sugar.

Refrigerator Staples

- **Unsweetened yogurt:** Unsweetened yogurt is the perfect blank canvas for a breakfast bowl. It allows you to control how much sweetener or sugar you add, which typically results in a lower-sugar meal than store-bought sweetened yogurt.
- **Whole milk:** I much prefer whole milk over skim milk because the fat content of whole milk makes it slightly more blood sugar–friendly.
- **Unsweetened plant-based milks:** Unsweetened plant-based milks, like almond milk or coconut milk, have a very low carbohydrate content and are great for dishes that already have a good amount of carbohydrates (like breakfast cereal or oatmeal), or when you want to add a creamer to your coffee but don't want to rely on sweetened options.
- **Berries:** Berries have one of the lowest glycemic indexes of any fruit, due to their naturally lower sugar content and higher fiber content compared to other fruits. They are great for adding a natural blood sugar–friendly sweetness to salads, smoothies, desserts, and more.

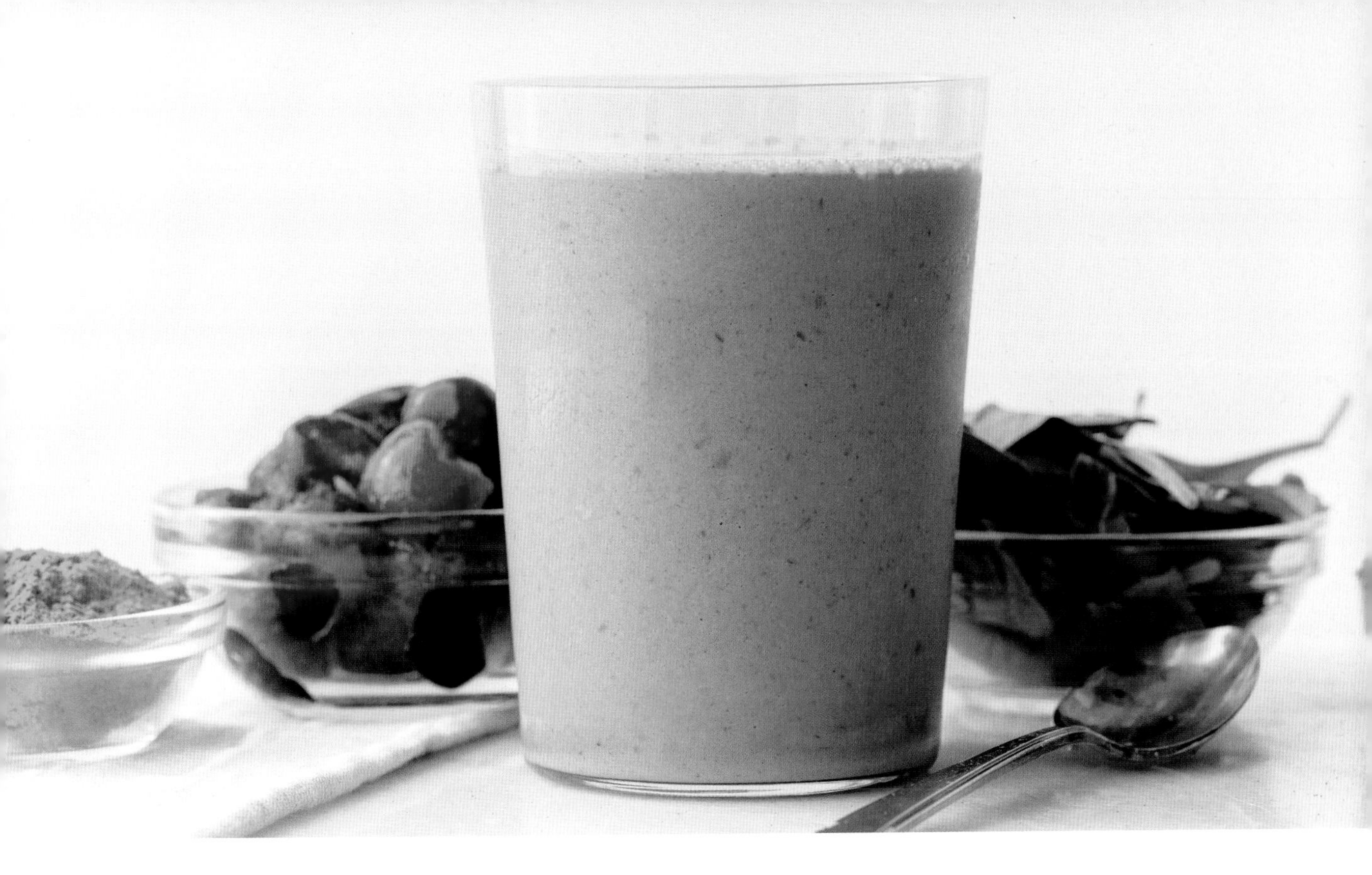

Kitchen Tools

- **Cookie scoop and ice cream scoop:** Cookie scoops and ice cream scoops come in standard sizes that can make measuring (and thus estimating carbohydrate counts) so much easier than having to get out measuring cups and spoons. I like to use them for portioning out batter or dough for baked goods, making pancakes, serving starchy dishes like potatoes, and more!
- **Zester:** Just like almond and vanilla extract, the zest from citrus fruits, especially lemons and oranges, can add so much flavor and sweetness to a dish without adding extra sugar.
- **Small food processor:** Most smaller food processors, many of which have a capacity of about 4 cups, will cost only about $30 and can be used for so many things in your kitchen to help you manage your blood sugars. I use mine for everything, from grinding up nuts to making small batches of homemade nut butter to blending fruit into unsweetened yogurt.

acknowledgments

Writing a cookbook has been my dream since I was a little girl, but there is no way I could have done this on my own. I want to thank the following people for never giving up on me . . .

My husband, Jason, for his constant love, encouragement, and willingness to taste test recipes.

My dad, for raising me to know I can do anything I set my mind to and instilling in me an entrepreneurial spirit that continually pushes me to dream big.

My mom, for constantly modeling to me when I was growing up that life with diabetes is not a death sentence, that it is manageable, and that you can live a perfectly normal and vibrant life with diabetes.

My grandmas, Mimi and Nette, for showing me how to bake and cook all the best dishes, from homemade cheesecake to chicken and dumplings.

My mother-in-law, for watching my girls at the drop of a hat when I needed time to write or test recipes.

Danielle Fineberg, for helping me develop, test, and fine-tune these recipes in the middle of a global pandemic that severely limited my time and suddenly had my kids at home with me.

Jenna at Page Street Publishing, for having enough faith in me to let me write a whole book and for always answering my questions, even when I felt silly or embarrassed.

Shay Paulson, for always being willing to be my second set of eyes on any content I produce, this book included.

Constance and Lauren of Studio Alcott, for their photography talent that far exceeded any expectations I ever could have had and for helping this book come to life.

Finally, to my daughters, for giving me a reason to constantly be better and dream big each and every day.

about the author

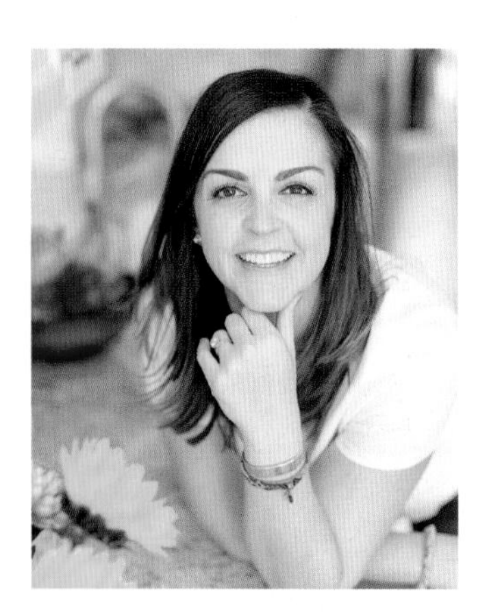

Mary Ellen Phipps is the founder and registered dietitian behind Milk & Honey Nutrition®. Mary Ellen has been living with type 1 diabetes since she was five years old, and she knows firsthand the impact food has on how we think, feel, act, and move. She strives to make food easy and fun again for people with diabetes. She uses both her professional expertise and personal experience to reduce stress and fear around food and to help people find joy in the kitchen. She lives in the Houston, Texas, area with her husband and two daughters.

Mary Ellen is also a contributing writer, recipe developer, and content expert for several leading health and wellness organizations. You can find her frequently on local Houston-area TV stations, educating audiences on food, nutrition, and joyful eating. She received a Bachelor of Science in Nutrition Sciences from Baylor University and a Master of Public Health in Epidemiology from the University of Texas School of Public Health.

index